the
nordic
diet

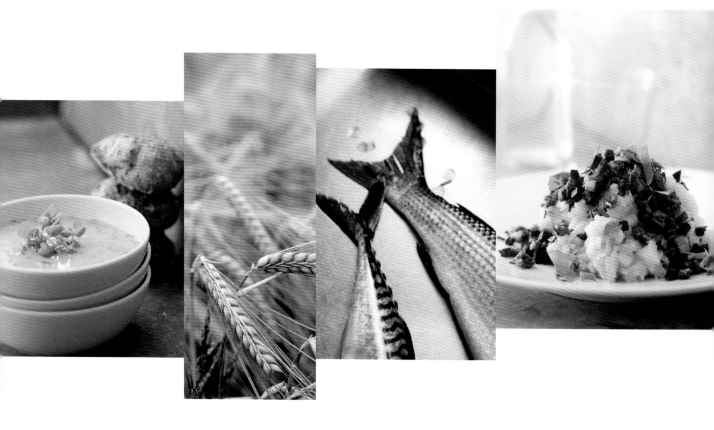

the nordic diet

Using Local and Organic Food to
Promote a Healthy Lifestyle

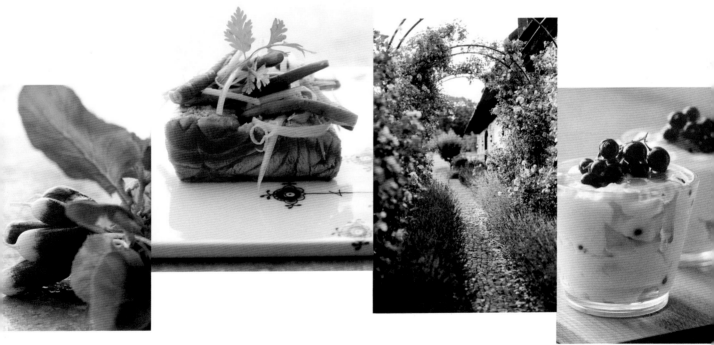

Trina Hahnemann

PHOTOGRAPHS BY LARS RANEK

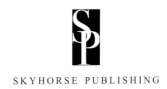

SKYHORSE PUBLISHING

To my mother Hanne Rodam
with thanks for all your support
and inspiration to do this book.

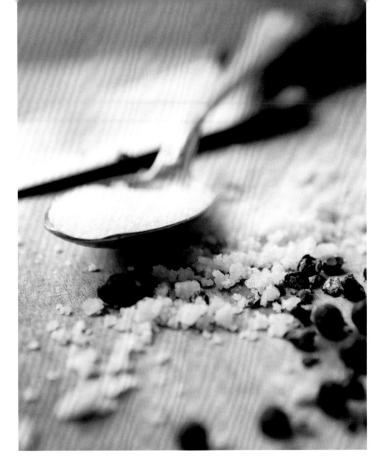

Foreword

After many years of advice concerning healthy food and eating being given on the basis of the Mediterranean diet, I am extremely pleased to introduce the Nordic diet as a meaningful alternative. It is a really healthy and sensible option for all of us who happen to live in the northern parts of this planet, and it can serve as an example for everybody everywhere interested in healthy food and living. Literally, it is like reaching out into your own backyard—all the produce is there to cook tasty, healthy Nordic food, beautiful dishes with kale, mackerel, cod, salmon, barley, spelt, oats, potatoes, horseradish, dill, and stinging nettles.

Ever since my childhood I have eaten good local produce introduced to me by my grandmother and parents. Then for some years I was led away from it by all kinds of foreign cuisines that seemed healthier choices with more flavors. For the last seven or eight years, though, I have gone back to my roots and cooked new and exciting recipes combined with elements from the cuisines of the world. I have found a very healthy way of living, by means of which I feel fit and can maintain my weight by eating good home-cooked food, which is seasonal, and where I really pay attention to what I buy, cook, and eat.

I cannot make myself eat strawberries out of season, because there is no joy in that. I'd much rather have them for three to five weeks a year and then really enjoy them, and when the season is over I will move on to the next seasonal thing. In many ways, I really believe your body needs that balanced diet, which good seasonal produce naturally provides.

The Nordic diet is also about cooking and eating habits: getting into the kitchen and cooking from fresh ingredients. Start baking your own bread! The most important thing about your diet, the way you eat, is that you should gain control over *what* you eat. You gain that by going into the kitchen and starting to cook. I cook three or four times a week and my husband will cook on the other days. We eat a lot of seasonal dishes and when we feel like a light meal we cook some pasta with seasonal vegetables, often using spelt or rye pasta, so it is about going back to your roots in a modern, healthy way.

Every evening we will be in the kitchen, which in my house is also an office, living room, and the place where I create all my recipes. We will be talking, our daughter doing her homework, her friends hanging out, our son coming by, neighbors dropping in, our lives being lived. And lives should be lived in the kitchen: cooking, baking, talking, eating, tasting, and being there together.

Take the time to get acquainted with the seasons and with what grows around you. Locate the markets nearby. What veg box schemes can you join? What could you grow yourself? And eat things that grow naturally around you. It does not have to be complicated. It is all about eating according to the season, cooking at home, appreciating what you eat, and taking time to enjoy life.

Velbekomme,

Trina Hahnemann

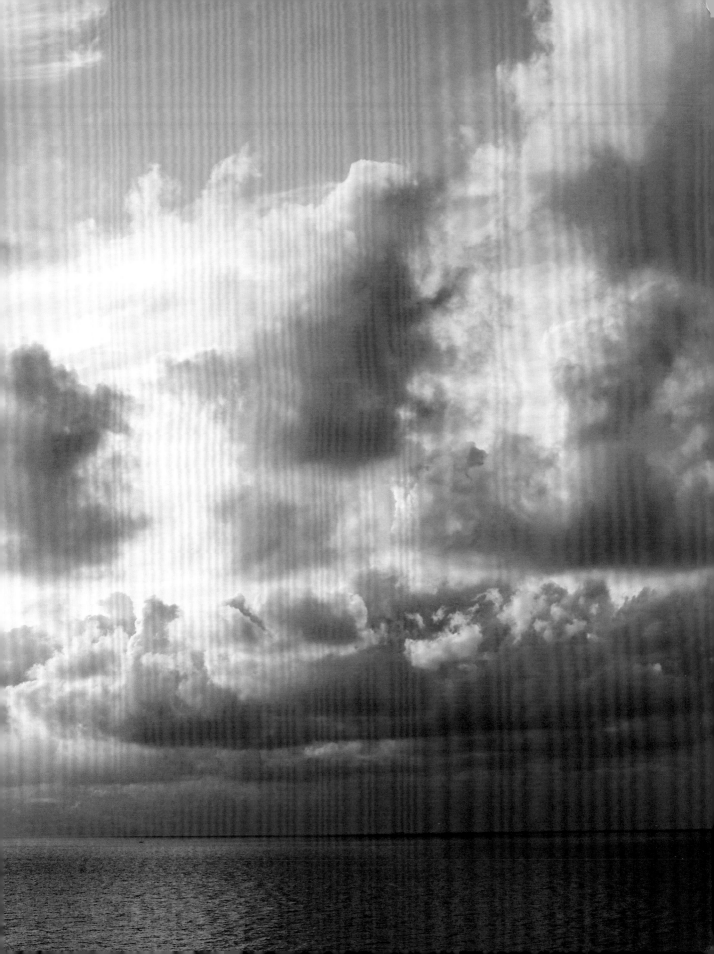

What Is the Nordic Diet?

The countries of the northern hemisphere have their own very healthy food culture, ingredients, and traditions which have, for too long, been eclipsed by the perceived benefits of the cuisines of other nations deemed to be intrinsically better for us. Rediscovering our Northern heritage also helps us address several issues around food other than health.

The fundamentals of the Nordic diet

- Balanced meals with an emphasis on whole grains and seasonal vegetables
- Home-cooking with fresh ingredients, including home-baked bread
- Eating less
- Eating fish at least twice a week
- Eating vegetarian meals twice a week
- Eating game, chicken, or meat only three times a week at most
- Taking time to eat with friends and family on a daily basis

The Nordic diet builds on tradition, but is also very much a modern, everyday cuisine incorporating influences from other cultures. It is based on the produce available in the northern hemisphere, where many grain and vegetable crops grow naturally or have ideal conditions for cultivation, where animals live wild or are farmed, and where fish that favor cold waters are caught or farmed.

Scientific evidence supports the claim that a balanced diet based on a wide base of ingredients with a variety of minerals, vitamins, beneficial fatty acids, and natural disease-fighting compounds will help you live a healthier and happier life. Of course, that alone is not enough. We also need to eat less—particularly of unhealthy foods like sugars and those full of saturated fats—and we need to get more exercise. Balance is at the core of a healthy and happy life.

The Nordic diet offers such a balance, with its focus on lots of different whole grains, root and green vegetables, locally caught fish and game, grass-fed lamb, and free-range poultry. It comes allied with a growing organic, eco-conscious movement and a focus on seasonality, so that during the year we dine more or less according to what nature has to offer.

The Nordic countries also offer a way of life that can positively add to the debate on the right balance between work, leisure, family time, and time spent cooking and eating. In Denmark, for instance, taxation makes cars so expensive that everyone cycles, to the great benefit of their fitness, their economy, and the air quality of Danish cities. In the Nordic countries we still cook a good deal and bake our own bread. Also, the evening meal is still a daily family event and that is an important part of being happy and healthy.

It is a myth that everything was better in the good old days. The food industry was not as developed as it is now and, faced with various socioeconomic problems, was not capable of feeding the population. Generally, there was not enough food, the diet was limited, vegetables and fruit were rare, and meat too expensive for average households. So when we consider all the problems today caused by the food industry, manifested in unrecognizable food that is full of additives, sugar, and salt, it becomes apparent that these are to some extent the result of circumstances in which it was necessary to produce food as efficiently and plentifully as possible.

These developments were also linked to the fact that many more women had entered the workforce, and generally nobody else volunteered to take over the cooking. This created a huge gap for the food industry to fill and our food culture suffered immensely.

This is, of course, a very short and generalized description of a highly complex problem, because there are a lot of important issues at stake here. However, I believe that, with the knowledge that we have today about health and obesity, we have to move forward and stop romanticizing the past. We have to decide on the food culture we want in the future and how we are going to lure people back into their kitchens: not to use their microwave oven to heat mass-produced convenience food but actually to cook food themselves from fresh ingredients; not buying bread made from grains that have been so refined that they have no taste or structure left, but making their own from nutritious and filling whole grains.

The Nordic diet is all about good, home-cooked food that is full of flavor, and about eating healthily without having to count calories all the time or obey strict dietary rules. It affords us an opportunity to change our diet according to local produce, seasons, tradition, and contemporary taste. Never before have the developed nations had access to so much food from all around the world; never has there been so much choice. However, in order to play our part in a sustainable global food culture for the future, we must now focus on our local cuisines, traditions, and produce. At this point in history we have an extraordinary opportunity to re-examine our daily food habits and, with our knowledge and technology, to develop a diet that encompasses different traditions with local produce.

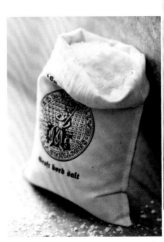
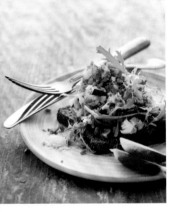

Diet & Lifestyle

Changing to a healthier lifestyle can be difficult, but the benefits are significant.

Change your diet

Your aim is to cook and eat food that is really tasty and full of fresh flavors that will give you joy and make you feel fulfilled and happy. This involves eating home-cooked meals, where love and care have been put into their preparation. Set the table, sit down, and enjoy the moment, eat slowly, and get your palate to work.

Take care to eat three main meals a day made up of whole grains, lots of tasty vegetables and fruit, and cut down on portion sizes. Your daily intake should be about 30–50 percent vegetables. In between meals you can snack on fresh or dried fruit, raw vegetables, and nuts. Keep your blood sugar levels in balance and don't starve yourself, but don't eat if you are not hungry.

Balance and variety are the key: Eat a balanced diet with lots of seasonal ingredients, while also making time for a piece of homemade cake or dessert now and then, a nice glass of wine, and eating more than you really should if you are having a good time eating with friends. Finding and keeping that balance is the key to a healthy and happy life.

Exercise more and spend time outside

It is important to understand that no matter how healthily you eat, exercise is still a key to health and happiness. Your heart is a muscle and it needs to be exercised, so cardiovascular exercise is good for your blood circulation, for your stress level, and for general psychological well-being, as well as to maintain a steady weight throughout

your life. If you don't exercise already, choose something you like—walking, swimming, running, cycling—something you will actually look forward to and enjoy doing. Start taking the stairs whenever you have the opportunity. Find other people to exercise with, set goals, or make a bet as an incentive to continue.

We have a saying in Denmark: "There is no such thing as bad weather, only wrong clothing." We bicycle a lot: to work, when we go shopping, and with our children. It's a great way to get around without being trapped in traffic. You do your bit for the environment, plus it is cheap and you get regular exercise built into your daily routine. If you can't cycle to work, get off one stop before your destination and walk the rest of the way.

We know vitamins, minerals, and antioxidants are important for the body's development and maintenance, but this is just one element of an overall balance in life. I therefore recommend living according to eight guidelines:

Eight guidelines to a healthier lifestyle

1. Exercise every day for at least thirty minutes.
2. Avoid junk food and ready-made meals; eat only things you know and recognize.
3. Eat at least six pieces of fruit and vegetables a day.
4. Eat whole grains in bread, cereals, salads, and pasta every day.
5. Reduce the fat in your food, especially dairy products and meat.
6. Eat fish two to three times a week.
7. Drink plenty of water.
8. Avoid sugar, especially in sodas, candies, cookies, and cakes.

Eat seasonal local produce

Another way to help the planet and to eat well is to buy meat, poultry, and dairy products from small or local farms. Buying organic or local food is a lifestyle in itself. No studies have yet proven that organic food is better for your health than nonorganically produced food, so eating organic is about what you believe is right. The main reason is to ensure that we do not over-exploit the earth and that we maintain an ecosystem without hormones, pesticides, and other chemicals that are difficult to recycle and harmful to the body.

Eggs from hens that find their food outside or from household leftovers taste better, and they improve results when baking. Cows from a farm where the farmers care about their pasture and the whole ecosystem, feeding their cows outside on good grass with clover, taste ten times better than cows produced in a shorter time frame on industrial feed. And to get really tasty seasonal vegetables: grow your own, join a veg box scheme, or buy at local stores and markets. Buy sustainable fish and support fairtrade products.

I support local buying, but I am also realistic. Coming from a Nordic country in which much food is not available locally all year round, we do need some supplies from other regions. Wine, coffee, and tea are prime examples of things that I would really miss if I could only buy food from a distance of up to 100 miles from where I live. Like everything else, it's all about finding a balance.

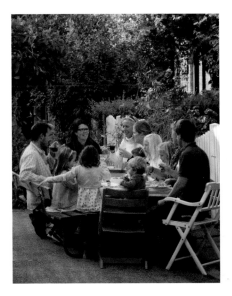

Eat meals together

Food must be a joy, not a burden, and this includes the social aspects of eating. I strongly believe it is immensely important to sit down regularly as a family to eat together. Eating with friends is also where you exchange life goals and life stories. Thinking about my dinner table and all the meals I've shared there with my friends, I recognize that it is an important part of my life: eating well-prepared food, talking, laughing out loud, crying, and enjoying all the stories told. It is also known that countries where food is prepared and shared have lower obesity rates.

Getting back into the kitchen, cooking healthy food from fresh ingredients, regularly setting a table nicely, and sitting down to share a meal—these are among the keys to healthy and happy living. I talk about this all the time, and the response I often get is: "We don't have time, we work late, and by the time everybody is home it's too late." Well, this is not necessarily true. You have plenty of time; you have a whole life full of time. Time is your capital; it is actually the most precious thing you have. The choice to be made is how to use that time. You have to ask: "Do you want a healthy life that includes two of the most important things for your body—proper food and exercise?" Then plan it to be so, and make a conscious decision that home-cooked food and eating together is part of your everyday life, and one thing you want to spend time doing.

Dealing with climate change

We all have to do our bit to help reduce climate change and global warming. Most of our attention is focused on travel, especially air travel and cars and their exhausts, but the world's livestock production is responsible for a large part of all greenhouse gases. The calculation is clear: It takes ten times more energy to produce a steak from a corn-fed cow than to produce the oats needed for a portion of oatmeal.

The solution is not only to return to grass-fed cows but to cut back drastically on the amount of meat we eat. So the modification of your diet is an area in which you can make a difference immediately: Stop eating meat every day; it's that simple. Cut down to a maximum of three times a week; your health will benefit, and you will do your bit to alleviate climate change. When you do buy meat spend more money on getting quality rather than on increasing the quantity.

One thing is sure: Driving a car to buy groceries every day is not good for the planet. Retrain yourself to shop only a couple of times a week or less, and walk or bicycle instead. But food transportation is also a complicated issue. We have established that for ecological and health concerns we need to cut down on meat consumption and eat more vegetables in our daily diet. The whole question of food mileage is very complicated, but I think one should be cautious about it: Do your own research and make your own judgment.

Small steps to fight global warming

- Reduce the amount of meat you eat.
- Buy as much food that's in season as possible.
- Choose locally grown fruit and vegetables that have not had to travel too far.
- Buy local fish, not exotic fish from the other side of the planet.
- Use your car as little as possible.

The Ingredients of the Nordic Diet

The Nordic diet is based around the indigenous produce of countries in the northern latitudes: whole grains, root and green vegetables, cold water fish and seafood, poultry and wild game, berries, and herbs. With only a few additions from other countries, these are all you need to provide a super-healthy balanced diet.

Grains

The grains used are those suited to cool climates—spelt, rye, oats, and barley, all of which are high in fiber and rich in protein. But beware, these are generally as refined and processed as most wheat flours, so it is vital to buy good-quality whole grains and whole-grain flours. Just as important is to bake for yourself, thereby avoiding mass-produced bread, which has little of the nutritive value of the grain and is full of additives to make it last. Never eat bread that is marked to last for more than a week.

Vegetables

Cabbages of all kinds—white, red, savoy, and pointed—together with their close relatives kale and Brussels sprouts, grow well in cold climates. They are low in calories, full of flavor, and can be cooked in many different ways. They have been found by scientists at the University of Oslo to contain some of the highest levels of antioxidants of any vegetable and are a good source of omega-3 fatty acids as well as vitamin K, which plays a role in blood coagulation. Moreover, they are full of phyto-chemicals strongly associated with anticancer action.

Root vegetables are also low in calories. At their seasonal best in fall and winter, they store well, and are versatile, filling, and fueling. Don't just stick with the usual potatoes and carrots: Try beet, celeriac, parsnips, parsley root, Jerusalem artichokes, and salsify, all of which are highly nutritious and tasty.

Green vegetables such as nettles, garlic, ramps (ramsons), Swiss chard, asparagus, peas, spinach, lettuce, and leeks provide us throughout the spring and summer with a wide range of nutrients and disease-fighting phytochemicals.

Fish and seafood

Fish from the cold northern waters are, of course, herrings, salmon, mackerel, and cod, but we also have wonderful lobster and crab, haddock, ling (cod), and monkfish, mussels, and oysters. They are all very healthy eating, low in calories and saturated fats but rich in protein and a wide range of nutrients.

Meat, poultry, and game

As with eggs, the flavor in meat, poultry, and game comes from the animal's diet. Animals that naturally feed in the wild, or are bred on pasture, generally have a better flavor than meat from animals reared in pens or stalls, unable to move and eating unnatural, commercial feed.

Chicken, and other poultry, is a very important source of protein, low in calories, and easy to prepare. However, a great deal of chicken nowadays is not so much raised as manufactured. You must be aware of the living conditions of the birds and what the creatures are fed on (both of which can be truly horrible), not only for their sakes but also because of what you are eating. I always buy free-range or organic chicken—more expensive, but our whole philosophy should be one of quality first, and reducing how much and how often we eat it.

Most game is seasonal and therefore forms an important part of fall eating, but you can get wild boar and some game birds all year round. Growing in the wild, game meat is healthier, leaner, and more digestible. If cutting down on meat intake, it makes sense to cut down on farmed meat and poultry and switch to wild game when it is in season.

Berries

Berries—blueberries and blackberries, red and black currants, rose hips, cloudberries (raspberries), lingonberries (cowberries)—are nature's free gift to us, growing wild in the countryside, ripe for picking. What is perhaps less well known is that research has now shown that they are among the healthiest foods we can eat, due to their ability to strengthen the human immune system and their high levels of antioxidants. The healthiest way to eat them is raw when in season, so take a walk in the woods, pick them fresh, and eat them as soon as you can.

Herbs

Herbs are immensely important in everyday cooking. Popular garden herbs include dill, parsley, chives, mint, tarragon, chervil, bay leaves, thyme, and rosemary. But we often forget the many wild herbs growing along our roadsides, such as horseradish and ground elder, considered as enemies by gardeners but full of health and taste. To get the most nutritional benefit from herbs you must eat large amounts, which you can do in soups and sauces, pestos, or salads like tabbouleh.

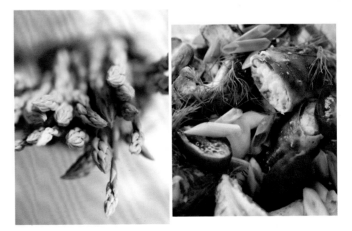

A Few Notes on Nutrition

I want to emphasize the properties of various foods and why they are good for you, so it might be helpful to provide some explanations of a few nutritional factors. You don't need to know all this, but it will make a useful reference to help you understand things more readily.

Antioxidants are molecules that prevent other molecules from oxidizing, i.e., combining with oxygen, a process that usually produces free radicals. In the body, such free radicals can be responsible for lots of health problems.

Carbohydrates are our source of energy from food. There are two types: complex and simple carbohydrates (or starches and sugars). The former come from foods like cereals, grains, and vegetables; the latter from sugar cane, vegetables like sugar beet, fruits, and honey. Complex carbs come with lots of other nutritional goodies, like dietary fiber, and provide a slow, steady source of energy. Simple carbs, on the other hand, generally offer little else but a quick jolt of energy that can cause the blood sugar level to climb rapidly and then collapse, causing you to feel hungry soon after eating them.

Cholesterol is a type of fat essential for the health of our cells. It is made by the body, but is also found in food. If we have too much of it in our blood it can form sticky deposits on our artery walls, which may build up and lead to strokes and heart disease. The body has mechanisms for controlling blood cholesterol levels, even if we eat large amounts of cholesterol-rich foods, like eggs, cheeses, meat, and shrimp. However, this process can be impaired by some health conditions and by an intake of too much saturated (animal) fats. There are two types of cholesterol, HDL and LDL, and it is too much of the latter that causes furring of the arteries, while the former actually helps clear the latter from the blood. Research has shown that blood HDL levels rise with activity and exercise.

Omega-3 and -6 fatty acids are also called essential fatty acids as they are the only fats the body needs but can't make itself. A good supply of them helps against all kinds of ailments, from heart disease and cancer to skin complaints. The average diet tends to provide more than enough omega-6s, but omega-3s, which act to reduce the stickiness of the blood, are harder to come by and are mostly found in oily fish . . . another reason to feast on fish.

Phytochemicals are compounds found in a wide variety of plants that don't provide nutrition but which actively help us fight disease. Many, and there are literally thousands, do this as they are antioxidants (see above) but others have the power to inhibit cancerous growth, lower levels of bad cholesterol in the blood, or actually thin the blood, and much more. These chemicals also tend to be those that give fruit and vegetables their characteristic colors, odors, and flavors. If nothing else, these are the reasons to eat your six-a-day . . . and more.

Protein is made from chains of amino acids and is essential for the body's growth and repair. Nowadays in developed countries we tend to get more than we need, as we only require about 0.4g a day per pound of body weight.

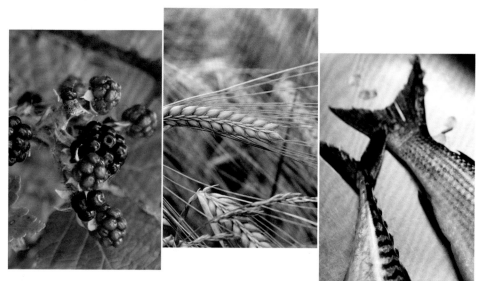

How to Lose Weight with the Nordic Diet

Losing weight—and keeping it off—can be hard work, because it involves life-changing decisions to find another way of eating and enjoying food. The rules couldn't be simpler, though: You need to burn more calories than you eat. Exercise is therefore vital. Being active means that you burn up more calories. At the same time, exercise improves your body's physical and mental state, so it is a win-win situation.

The average recommended calorie intake for women to maintain their body weight is 2,000 calories a day; for men it is 2,500 calories. To lose 2 pounds per week you need to lower your daily calorie intake by 500 calories OR significantly increase your activity level. However, increased activity levels make you hungrier, so I would recommend a balance of both.

I have to emphasize that this is a general guideline. The metabolism varies from individual to individual, depending on age, gender, height, weight, and your everyday activity levels. Furthermore, if you exercise regularly, the proportion of heavier muscular tissue to fat changes. I recommend that you consult a nutritionist or dietitian to have your personal calorie needs determined more precisely.

The most important thing about weight loss is to change your lifestyle forever . . . and I mean forever. I can't recommend going on a diet for two to three weeks and then going back to eating like you used to. That way you can't expect to keep the pounds off; moreover, such "yo-yo" dieting can be very damaging to your health. Changing your lifestyle is crucial if you need to lose weight and maintain your new body weight. That means smaller portions and less food, more vegetables and complex carbs, less alcohol, fat, and sugar—and some exercise every day.

It is actually that simple and can be done without calculating anything. I don't mean you can't indulge yourself ever again; I'm all for having fun, wonderful food, and nice wine. I am talking about changing your habits and your palate, so you end up preferring real-tasting food that is good for you. The positive side of being on a diet is that it takes up a short period of time compared with your whole lifespan.

Ground rules before starting a diet

Before you start your diet make a decision that these are changes that are going to be a permanent part of your life from now on. After some months without a lot of the things you are used to, such as potato chips, french fries, sodas, sugar in everything, heavy sauces, etc., they will actually lose their appeal . . . I promise. Real flavors from real food can really change your preferences!

Take time planning and cooking: Eating on the move is not a good solution, and shopping for food when you are very hungry and your blood sugar levels are low is also a bad idea. Therefore, plan three to four days ahead or maybe even for a whole week.

Eating together at a set table is important—don't eat in front of the TV!

Make sure your dinner plates are not too big; using smaller plates is a good way to control portion sizes.

Eat all your meals slowly, enjoy your food, and taste it—I mean really taste it and focus on what's on your palate. Learning to eat slowly can be hard in the beginning; I know from my own experience. At the beginning I put my watch next to the plate to keep track of time, and promised myself that the eating had to take at least thirty minutes. It took me a couple of months really to get into the habit.

Involve other people for support. If you find it difficult to change your habits, tell them how they can help you to achieve your goals.

Establishing your ideal weight

Your ideal weight is an individual matter. A good guideline is body mass index (BMI). Most governments use this indicator in the assessment of public health, which is fine, but, again, individual circumstances should be taken into account. You can use the formula below or, even easier, you will find BMI calculating pages online and all you have to do is tap in your height and weight and they will calculate your BMI for you.

BMI = $\dfrac{705 \times \text{body weight in pounds}}{\text{height in inches} \times \text{height in inches}}$

BMI	Status
Below 18.4	Underweight
18.5 – 24.9	Normal
25 – 29.9	Overweight
30 & above	Obese

Planning your weight-loss diet

Start your new diet by examining everything in your cupboards, getting rid of not-very-healthy convenience items, such as ready meals, canned soups, snack bars, milk chocolate, sodas, potato chips, cereals containing sugar, and so on. Then restock your cupboards with real food, good oils and vinegars, whole grains, oats, and flours. This replacement process can, of course, be rather expensive. If so, you can do it over time, but try to get rid of all the unhealthy choices in your cupboards as quickly as possible. That is the surest way not to be tempted to eat them.

Plan what to eat for the whole week ahead, and then only go shopping twice so that you spend time in the kitchen instead of in the stores. When on a diet, planning is the key to success. Shopping when hungry or on the spur of the moment will almost inevitably mean that the wrong things get in your basket.

Make sure you always have vegetables and fresh and dried fruits and nuts in the house, so when you get really hungry or fatigued you have something safe to eat.

High days and vacations

Vacations are always exceptions, and it is only natural to gain a little weight after a couple of weeks with good food and wine every day. That is OK and part of life, but make sure you exercise and perhaps increase your activity level while you have time on your hands.

If you go to a party or have a day when you get lunch with friends, or any event where your calorie intake is higher than planned, just cut down on the following days and you will still lose the amount you need for that week. Dieting is a process that cannot be evaluated day by day but only over weeks or months.

Salt

Sodium is an essential mineral that we mostly get from salt. Unfortunately, getting too much salt is linked with risk of high blood pressure and heart disease. Your average intake should not be higher than 6g per day. Weigh it up and see how much that is—that will give you a clear picture of the amount and help you limit it. To avoid too much salt in your diet, do not eat processed food, takeout and lots of cookies and snacks bars, as they contain a lot of salt because it is a natural flavor enhancer. Cut back on added salt when cooking; let people add it if necessary.

Sugar

Over the last few decades sugar has become the big enemy, but not because there is anything wrong with sugar; gastronomically it is a fantastic ingredient and I would not live without it. However, consuming sugar in the quantities we do is a real and threatening problem, leading to all sorts of health concerns from obesity and acne to diabetes and hormone imbalances.

Stop using sugar in your tea and coffee, but do not replace it with any sweetener. Instead, get used to the true taste of the coffee and tea. Do this in stages if necessary. Stop drinking soda on a daily basis and, instead, buy or make some organic cordials and dilute them with water. Stop eating snack bars, chocolate bars, store-bought cakes, and cookies and candies. When craving sweet things, bake yourself a cake (NOT using a ready-made cake mix) so you control exactly what goes into the cake—that is, the quantity of sugar and the quality of the other ingredients. Eat fruit instead. Even though it also contains sugar, it is still a healthy option.

What should you aim for?

If you want to lose weight in a healthy and steady way, I recommend losing 1–2 pounds a week, no more. Then you will then not starve or feel fatigued. The weight loss will all be due to change. Be patient if nothing really happens in the beginning; just stick to it, and the weight will eventually start coming off.

When you have to lose weight, it is important to maintain a steady blood-sugar level. You do that by eating six meals a day: three main ones and three small ones. The diet plan (opposite) will work if you do not sit still all day but move around 20 percent of the time, and exercise two to three times a week.

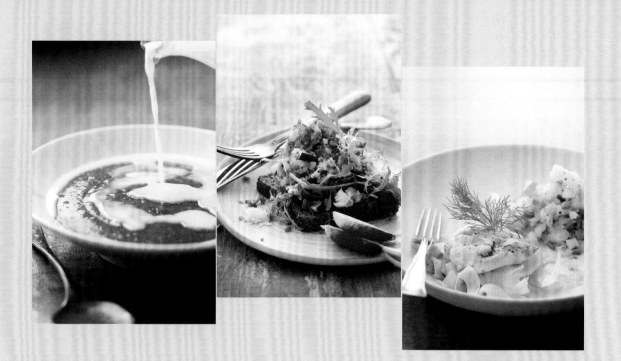

Day's model diet plan for losing weight

Breakfast
1 portion of raw oats with fruit and nonfat skim milk, or oatmeal, or a piece of rye bread with cottage cheese (see the recipes on pages 22–27).
Coffee or tea* (with no sugar).

Morning snack
A snack between breakfast and lunch is important to make sure you don't get tempted to grab something unhealthy to fill the gap.
1 piece of rye bread with 2 tablespoons of low-fat cottage cheese, or if at a desk far from a kitchen, have some raw vegetables and ⅓ oz nuts, like walnuts, hazelnuts, or almonds.

Lunch
A standard lunch with pieces of rye bread with hard-boiled eggs, or potatoes (see page 39) and a portion of raw vegetables like carrots, cauliflower, cucumber, or celery stalks. On weekends or at home, when you have more time and a kitchen is available, make soup or some of the other lunch recipes in the book.

Afternoon snack
1 piece of fruit.

Dinner
1 piece of fish, poultry, or game, about 5 oz (except for days where the meal is vegetarian).
1 big portion of vegetables.
2 potatoes or 1 piece of whole-grain bread
1 portion of salad, with lettuce, kale, or cabbage.

Choose from the recipes in the book:
Divide each week as follows:
three days with fish**
two days with vegetarian meals
two days with meat.

When having your main meal, make sure you set the table nicely, prepare your food with love, and take time eating at the table with your family or friends; if eating alone, still set the table and serve yourself a wonderful, tasty dinner.

Eat only one portion of food, then eat slowly and drink plenty of water while eating. That also prolongs the meal.

Always serve a fresh salad according to the season; fresh raw vegetables fill you up and they are low in calories. When on a diet, avoid dressings; instead, use lemon juice or a nicely flavored quality vinegar instead.

In general, cut down on fat. Steam or bake instead of pan-frying.
** If you have an allergy and can't eat fish, have meat instead.

Evening snack
⅔ cup nonfat yogurt with berries or other seasonal fruit or, some nights, a small piece of dark chocolate.

General
Drink 8 cups of water a day, and always have raw vegetables in a plastic bag to snack on if hungry or getting sugar cravings.
*Coffee and tea are unlimited, but be careful not to have too much caffeine, which can make you hyper, especially if you do not eat a lot. Always use skim milk in your coffee and tea. Avoid café latte, as there are too many calories in all that milk, and that goes for soy latte as well.

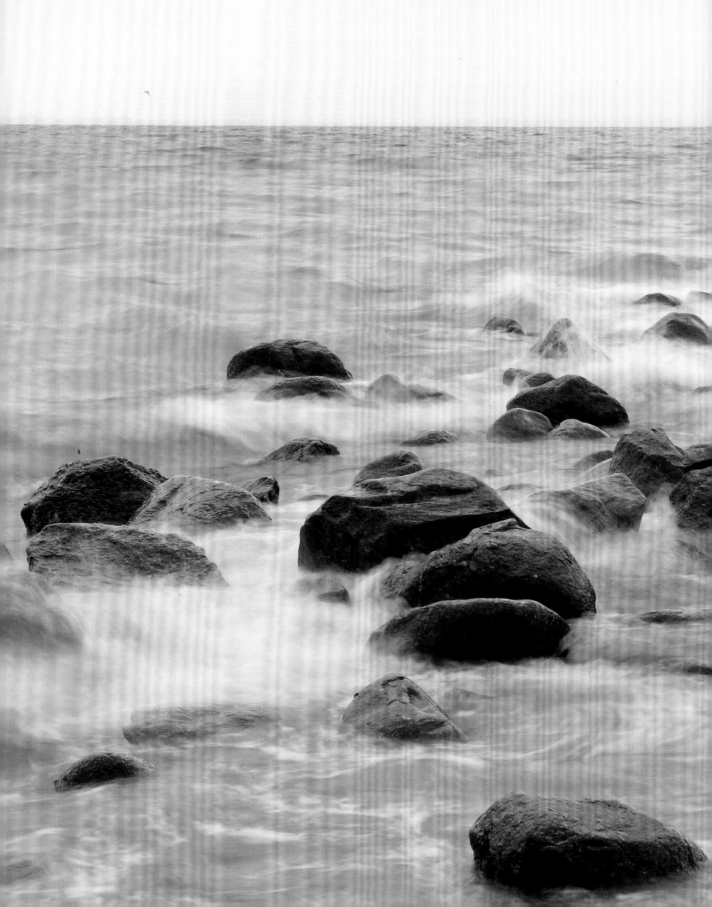

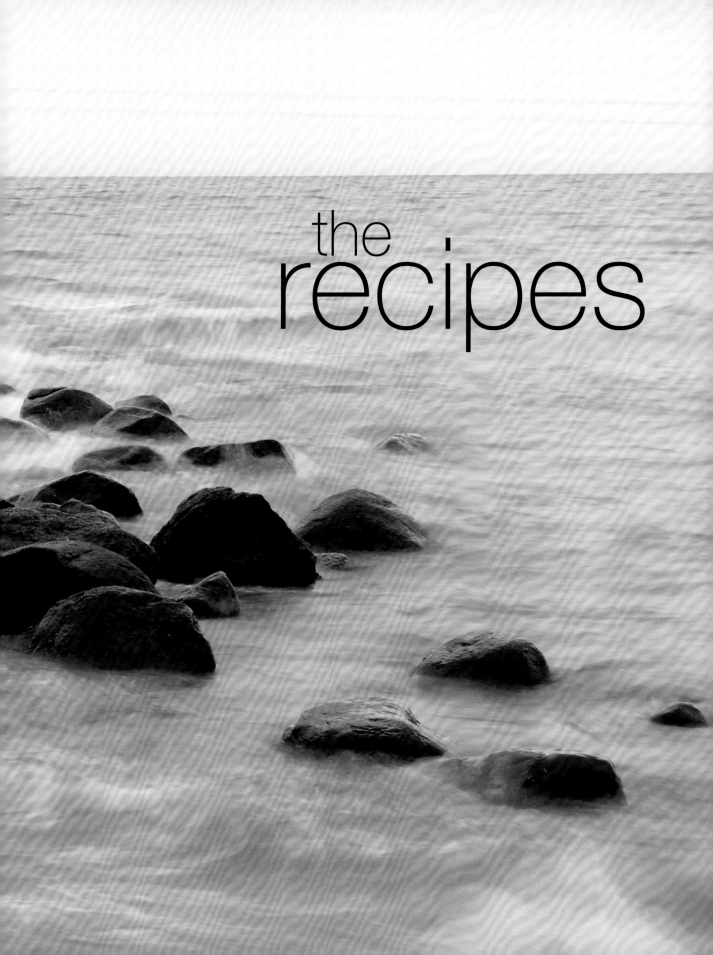

the
recipes

Breakfast

Breakfast is a very important meal; in fact, most nutritionists consider it THE most important meal of the day. A healthy, balanced breakfast, with a good content of complex carbohydrates, gives you a better start to the day, particularly in the case of children. It is therefore important not to make it a meal of white bread or sugary cereals, because these will not give you sufficient energy that will last the morning. Instead, have something hearty, like whole grains, fruit, vegetables, and eggs, which will keep hunger at bay at least until lunchtime.

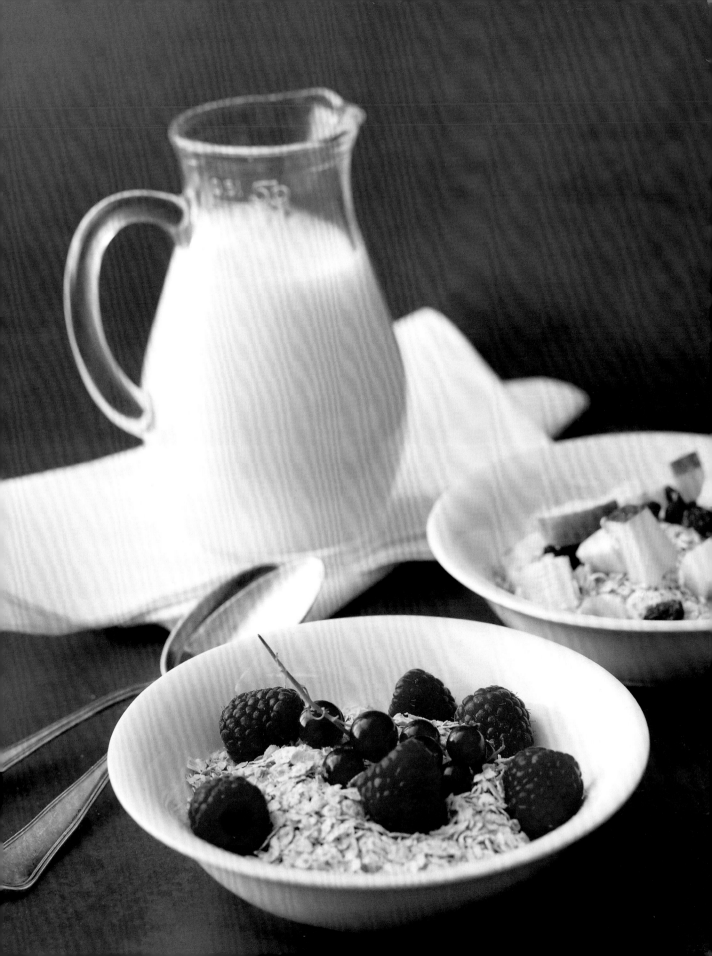

Raw oats with fruit and milk in summer

(illustrated on previous page)

This was my breakfast throughout childhood—and I would also have raw oats with milk and sugar as a snack after school (snack bars were not as readily available then as they are today). My children also grew up on this and have both grown to be tall and healthy, although they often complain, as they believe that if they hadn't had all these organic oats, fruit, and the organic skim milk, then they would have been more like everybody else! SERVES 1

scant 1 cup raw rolled oats
½ cup red currants
6 raspberries
generous ¾ cup skim milk

Add the oats to a serving bowl as a little mountain in the middle. Place the fruit around the oats, pour the milk over everything, and eat right away.

VARIATION For a winter version of this, you can replace the berries with ½ cup diced apple and a generous ⅛ cup seedless raisins.

TIP The rolled oats can be replaced with 2 WeetaBix.

Smoothies

These make super fast and very healthy breakfasts as they contain lots of the "superfoods." All sorts of smoothies can easily be made, you just need a blender, frozen or fresh fruit, fruit juice, or low-fat yogurt, and some honey. Then mix these any way you like to create your favorite smoothie.

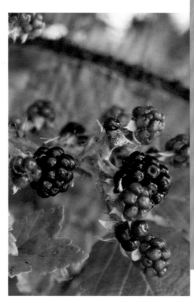

Berries of all types contain large amounts of antioxidant vitamins A and C. The blueberry contains the most antioxidants of sixty of the most common berries and vegetables, as well as omega-3 fatty acids. Blueberries and mulberries grow wild and are cultivated throughout most of Europe and the United States. Blackberries are one of the few fruits to contain significant amounts of antioxidant vitamin E, and they also contain the phytochemical ellagic acid, which may block several types of cancer.

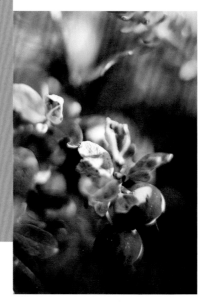

Red currant smoothie
SERVES 2

2 cups fresh or frozen
    red currants
1 banana, peeled
generous ⅓ cup red currant cordial
1¼ cups low-fat yogurt
honey, to sweeten (optional)
handful of ice cubes (if using
    fresh fruit)

Place all of the ingredients into
a blender and blend. Taste and
sweeten with honey if you like.
Serve right away in tall glasses.

Blueberry smoothie
SERVES 2

2 cups blueberries
generous ⅓ cup apple juice
1 banana, peeled
1¼ cups low-fat yogurt
10 ice cubes
honey, to sweeten (optional)

Place all of the ingredients into a
blender and blend. Taste and adjust
the sweetness with some honey if you
like. Serve right away in tall glasses.

Strawberry and raspberry smoothie
SERVES 2

2 cups fresh or frozen strawberries
    and raspberries
1 banana, peeled
generous ⅓ cup orange juice
generous 2 cups low-fat yogurt
honey, to sweeten (optional)
handful of ice cubes (if using
    fresh fruit)

Place all of the ingredients into a
blender and blend. Taste and
sweeten with honey if you like.
Serve right away in tall glasses.

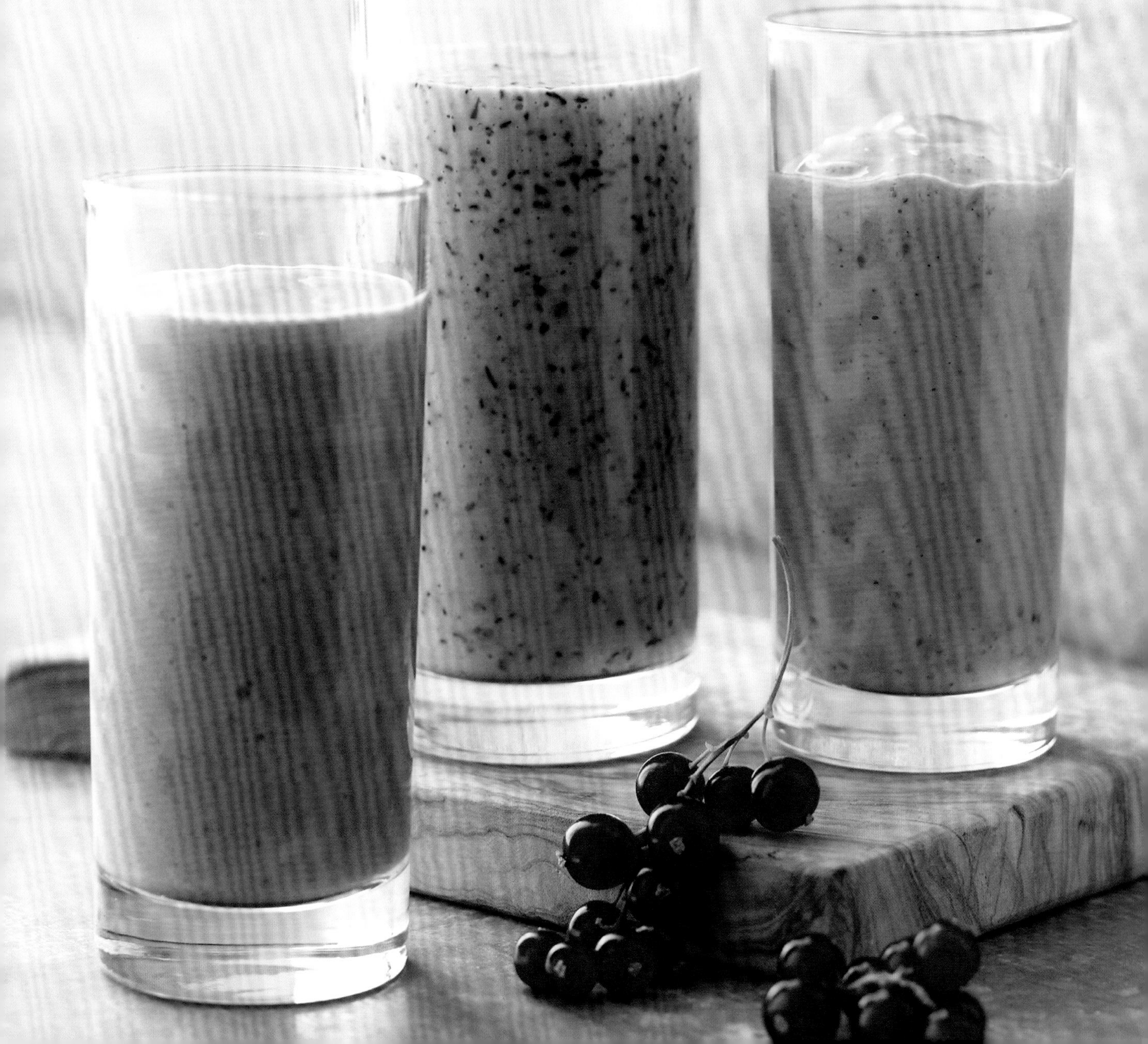

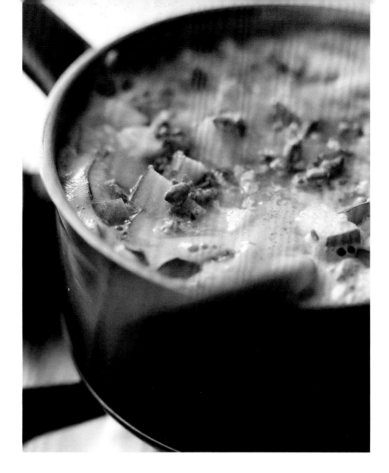

Fruity morning oatmeal

The grains here all have a low GI, so they provide energy all morning, and are packed full of other goodies. Rye and spelt are rich in minerals and vitamins B1 and B3, while oats are particularly healthy as they are also rich in beta-glucans, which reduce blood cholesterol levels. Only a hundred years ago families frequently ate all kinds of oatmeal for their evening meal because their means did not allow them to have meat and vegetables every day. I believe it would be a good idea for our climate, health, and wallets if we took up eating oatmeal again as a main course during the week. SERVES 4

3 oz rye flakes
2 oz spelt flakes
3 oz whole oat flakes
¼ cup raisins
1 apple, about 3½ oz, cored and diced
1½ tsp salt flakes
cold skim milk, to serve

Mix all the grains in a bowl and place them in a pan with the raisins, apple, and 4 cups of water. Bring to a boil, lower the heat, and let simmer for 5–8 minutes. Season with salt. Serve the oatmeal right away and very hot with some cold skim milk.

TIP I buy big bags of the grains and then I mix them and keep them in a jar. For one portion, I use 2½ oz of the grain mix, add my fruit and raisins, then cook and simmer it as above.

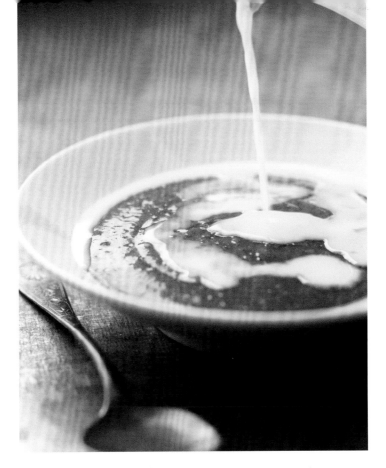

Rye and beer oatmeal

This very traditional Nordic oatmeal made from leftover rye bread was eaten for the evening meal. I love to have it for breakfast in the winter. SERVES 4

11 oz rye bread that is a couple
   of days old
1 tsp grated lemon zest
generous ¾ cup light or alcohol-free beer
½ cup brown sugar
cold skim milk, to serve

The day before, place the bread in a bowl, cover with 3⅓ cups water, and leave overnight.

The next day, place the contents of the bowl in a pan and slowly bring to a boil. Stir well, add the lemon zest, beer, and sugar, boil, and keep stirring for 5 minutes.

Serve warm with cold skim milk.

TIP You can serve this as a dessert with whipped cream.

Spelt pancakes with blueberries

Spelt has a sweet taste. I think the flour is perfect for pancakes and some cakes, but it is difficult to bake without adding a little all-purpose flour, as there is very little gluten in spelt flour, and gluten is what makes the dough elastic, helping it to rise. SERVES 4 OR 6 (12 PANCAKES)

2 eggs
1¾ cups buttermilk
1 vanilla bean
scant 1½ cups spelt flour
scant ¾ cup all-purpose flour
1 tsp baking soda
1 tsp salt
scant 2¼ cups fresh blueberries
6 tbsp butter, for cooking
runny honey or syrup, to serve

To make the pancake batter, beat the eggs together in a large mixing bowl. Add the buttermilk and beat again. Split the vanilla bean lengthwise and scrape out the seeds with the tip of a knife. Mix the vanilla seeds, flours, baking soda, and salt together, then add to the egg mixture and beat again until smooth. Mix in 1 cup of the blueberries.

Melt a little butter in a skillet and, using a soup spoon, place three separate spoonfuls in the skillet so that you cook three small round pancakes at a time, gently turning them once, until nicely browned on both sides. Keep each batch warm under a dishtowel while you cook the rest.

Serve right away, topped with more fresh blueberries and honey or syrup. TIP If you want to lose weight, eat one pancake with ⅔ cup fruit as your weekend treat, but don't add any honey or syrup.

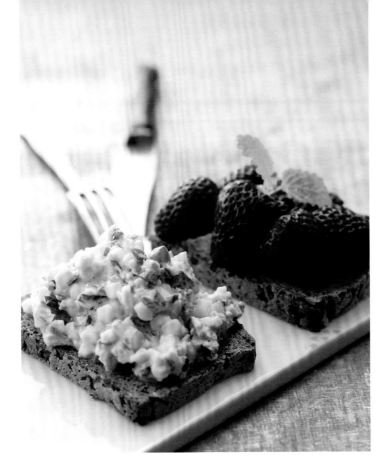

Rye bread madder (open sandwiches)

These easy and healthy breakfast ideas also make perfect snacks at any time during the day. If you are aiming to lose weight, it is very important to eat small meals during the day so that your blood sugar levels do not drop drastically, causing you to go for a high-sugar quick fix like a chocolate bar. In the strawberry season, the perfect afternoon snack is a strawberry "madder," a piece of rye bread with a very simple topping. SERVES 2

Rye bread with strawberries

generous 1⅓ cups strawberries
2 slices of rye bread

Cut the strawberries in half, then place them on rye bread and eat right away.

   VARIATION Mash some raspberries gently and spread out evenly on a piece of rye bread like jam, and you have the perfect summer "mad."

Rye bread, cottage cheese, herbs, and vegetables

scant 1 cup cottage cheese
2 tbsp chopped chives
2 tomatoes, seeded and diced
⅓ cucumber, halved, seeded, and diced
salt flakes and freshly ground pepper
2 slices of rye bread

Place the cottage cheese in a bowl and mix with the other ingredients except the seasoning and the bread. Season to taste with salt and pepper. Place on top of the slices of rye bread and serve right away.

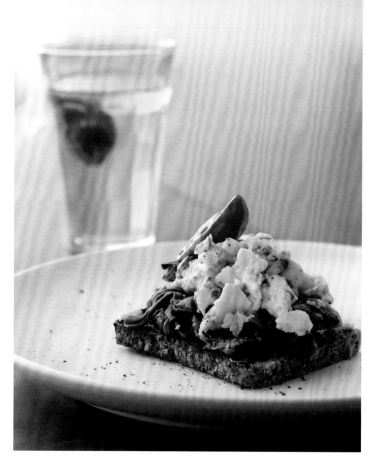

Eggs on rye toast with spinach

Eggs are highly nutritious, a great source of protein and have a low GI, so they give you long-burning energy all morning. Until quite recently eggs were rather demonized by healthy eating campaigners as they have quite a high cholesterol content, but nutritionists now feel that this is outweighed by their plus points, and that eggs pose no threat to those who don't have problems with high blood cholesterol levels. Ten a week is a good limit—and this includes eggs in baked goods like cakes and cookies, as well as in sauces. SERVES 4

2¼ lbs fresh spinach
salt and freshly ground pepper
4 slices of rye bread
8 organic eggs
¼ cup skim milk
1 tbsp canola oil
10 wild garlic leaves, or
  chives, or scallion greens,
  chopped
10 cherry tomatoes, diced

Start by preparing the spinach: Remove any tough stems from the leaves and rinse three or four times in cold water. Drain in a colander.

Wilt the spinach in a sauté pan for 3 minutes. Season with salt and pepper, then drain in a colander again.

Put the bread to toast.

Mix the eggs in a bowl, beat them for 1 minute, then beat in the milk. Season the mixture. Add the oil to the sauté pan, heat gently then pour the egg mixture into the pan. Add the leaves, chives, or greens, lower the heat, and cook gently. Just before the eggs start to set, add the tomatoes.

Place a slice of rye toast on each plate, divide the spinach between them, then add the eggs, sprinkle with pepper, and serve right away.

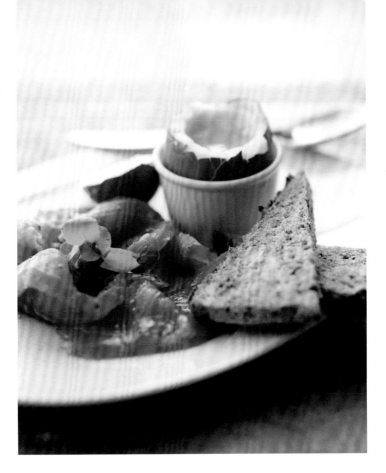

Soft-boiled egg with toasted rye bread and smoked salmon

During weekends, when we have enough time to enjoy a long breakfast, I cook a meal that is more time-consuming and eat it with my husband while we take our time reading the newspapers. Soft-boiled eggs are a real treat, are easy to digest, and give a fantastic boost to start your metabolism in the morning. SERVES 2

2 large organic eggs
2 slices of rye bread
4 slices of smoked salmon
a little handful of watercress

Place the eggs in a small pan with just enough cold water to cover. Bring to a boil, lower the heat, and let it simmer gently for 3 minutes.

While the eggs are cooking, toast the rye bread and place the salmon on a small plate. Place the watercress on top of that and sprinkle with pepper. When the eggs are cooked, rinse them under cold running water. Drain and place them in egg cups.

Serve with the smoked salmon and rye bread on the side.

TIP Cooking eggs is a mystery. It takes training and concentration, and it is unbelievable that something so simple goes wrong so often. Often—and therefore most likely—we don't know how old our eggs are, and fresh eggs take a bit longer to cook than those that are a week old. The size of the eggs also matters. All in all, if you are a newcomer to the art of boiling eggs, just practice and you will eventually learn.

Light Lunches

Ensuring you get a healthy lunch is usually a bit of a problem as we often have to rely on what other people have cooked for us, or on what we can buy. When we buy ready-made meals, they often contain a lot of calories, salt, sugar, or additives—all the stuff we would like to avoid in a healthy lifestyle. Lunch, therefore, needs planning. Get the most out of your vegetables by preparing soups and salads. Having a tasty smooth soup followed by a crunchy salad makes a very satisfying and healthy meal.

Baked fish and parsley pesto sandwich

This is a simple but good sandwich for lunch. The shower bun dough (page 131) is very suitable to make into big flat sandwich bread for this sandwich. Parsley is a rather overlooked healthy food, rich in iron, carotenoids, and vitamin C. It is also known to aid liver and/or gallbladder function. SERVES 2

14 oz skinless fish fillets
salt and freshly ground pepper
2 spelt or rye buns
3½ oz fresh salad greens
2 tomatoes, sliced

parsley pesto
1 large bunch of parsley
scant ¼ cup almonds (with their skins)
1 small garlic clove, chopped
3 tbsp freshly grated
   Parmesan cheese
3 tbsp grapeseed oil
juice from 1 unwaxed lemon
salt and freshly ground pepper

Preheat the oven to 400°F. Start by making the pesto: Put all of the ingredients except the lemon juice, salt, and pepper into a blender, and blend to a smooth paste. Season to taste with lemon juice, salt, and pepper.

Place the fish fillets in an ovenproof dish, sprinkle with salt and pepper, and bake in the oven for 10 minutes.

Cut the buns in half and spread some pesto on both halves of each, then place some salad on that, then the baked fish, and then the tomatoes.

Serve with the fish either warm or cold.

TIP Save the rest of the pesto for a salad, or serve it with a piece of broiled fish or chicken breast.

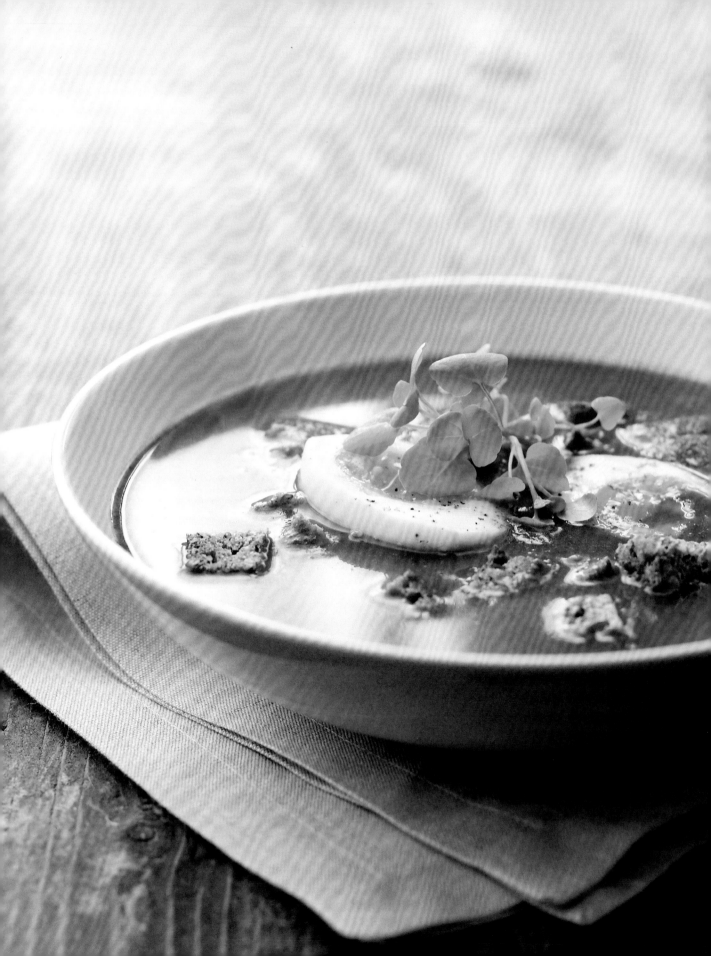

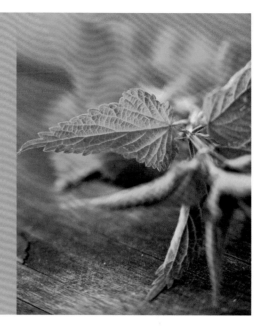

STINGING NETTLES are an old medicinal herb and their stems have been used for weaving textiles since at least the Bronze Age. It grows everywhere in the countryside where the soil contains a certain level of nitrogen. The stinging nettle is a king among herbs, as it is extremely rich in vitamins A, C, and D, and in iron, potassium, manganese, calcium, and silicon, which is good for the bones and healthy for the skin. It also contains high levels of vegetable protein. Cooking or drying completely neutralizes the plant's toxic components. It must be picked in spring and early summer before flowering.

Stinging nettle soup

Stinging nettle soup should be made in May, when the stinging nettle has a lot of top leaves. Pick only the four or five top leaves. Nettle leaves are also good in scrambled eggs and frittatas—just blanch the leaves before use. SERVES 4

1 yellow onion
1 tbsp olive oil
5½ cups organic vegetable bouillon
¼ tsp ground nutmeg
7 oz stinging nettles (see above)
salt and freshly ground pepper
a few sprigs of watercress, to serve
4 organic eggs, to serve

garlic croutons
2 slices of rye or spelt bread, cut
  into cubes
1 tbsp olive oil
1 garlic clove, minced
salt and freshly ground pepper

First make the croutons: Preheat the oven to 350°F. Mix the bread cubes with the oil, garlic, salt, and pepper, and bake in the oven for 10 minutes.

In a large pan, sauté the onion in the oil for 5 minutes without allowing it to burn or color too much. Add the vegetable bouillon and nutmeg, bring to a boil, and add the nettle leaves. Let simmer for 20 minutes.

Using a hand blender, blend the soup, then season with salt and pepper.

Bring some water to a boil in a small pan. When the water is boiling, place the eggs in the water, turn down the heat, and let simmer for 7 minutes. Remove from the heat and place under cold water for 30 seconds. Take out and shell right away.

Serve the soup with the boiled eggs cut across in half and the croutons and watercress scattered on top.

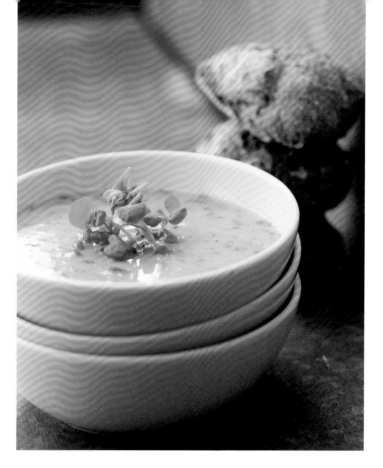

Cold cucumber soup

On a very hot summer's day, when you don't really have a big appetite, serve this clear, fresh, tasty soup. SERVES 4

1 tsp canola oil
2 scallions, sliced
2 cucumbers, halved,
  seeded, and diced
generous 2 cups yogurt
2 tbsp chopped mint
salt and freshly ground pepper
a few sprigs of watercress, to serve
spelt bread (page 138), to serve

chicken stock

1 chicken, about 2¼ lbs
2 tsp salt
1 tbsp whole peppercorns
1 bay leaf

First make the stock: Place the chicken in a pot, pour over scant 3¼ quarts water, and add the salt, pepper, and bay leaf. Bring to a boil and let simmer for 1 hour, removing as much scum as possible from the surface. Remove the chicken and save for a salad or something else. Strain the stock through a strainer and let cool until lukewarm.

Add the oil to a large pan and then add the scallions. Sauté for 5 minutes, but do not let them turn brown, only golden. Add 4 cups of the chicken stock, bring to a boil, turn off the heat, and add the cucumber.

Using a food processor, blend to a creamy soup.

Let the soup cool down completely. Add the yogurt and the chopped mint, and season with salt and pepper.

Garnish with watercress and serve with spelt bread.

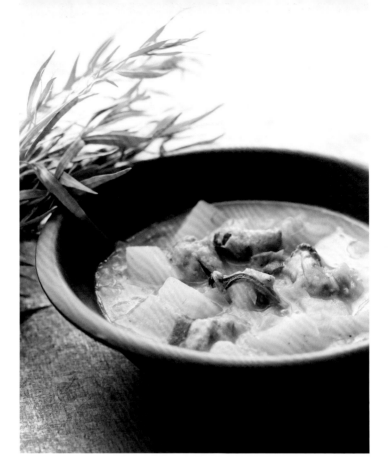

Mussel soup with potatoes and leeks

New England clam chowder is one of my favorite soups, but it is very high in calories. Here is my Nordic version, which has fewer calories but is still very tasty. SERVES 4

2¼ lbs mussels
1 tbsp canola oil
1 onion, minced
2 garlic cloves, chopped
3 leeks, cut into slices
1 tbsp tarragon leaves
salt and freshly ground pepper
4 large potatoes, peeled and diced
spelt baguettes (page 137), to serve

Scrub the mussels thoroughly and tug out any beards that may be hanging from the shells. Discard broken or open mussels or those that refuse to close when tapped. Rinse the mussels in water a couple of times.

Heat the oil in a big pan. Add the onion, garlic, and leeks, and cook for 3 minutes. Add the mussels with the tarragon, 4 cups of water, and salt and pepper. Bring to a simmer and let simmer for 15 minutes.

Take out the mussels with a slotted spoon. Remove the mussels from the shells and discard the shells. Take out a generous ¾ cup of the soup and place in another pan. Add 2 of the diced potatoes to that and let it simmer for 15 minutes.

To the large pot with the soup add the shelled mussels with the juice and the leeks that came out with the mussels. Add the rest of the potatoes and let simmer for 15 minutes.

Blend the potato soup in the small pan with a hand blender until it is a smooth, heavy soup, then add it back to the main soup and heat it up. Season to taste with salt and pepper.

Serve the soup very hot with spelt baguettes.

Leek soup with rye croutons

This nourishing soup is easy to make and very inexpensive. I believe that eating vegetable soup for the evening meal once a week is a good way to organize your diet, giving you a day without meat, a day where you save money, and a day when your supper is healthy and fiber-intensive. SERVES 4

1 tbsp canola oil
1 shallot, diced
2 garlic cloves, chopped
1 tsp ground cardamom
5 leeks, well rinsed and cut
  into slices
3 bay leaves
6⅓ cups organic vegetable bouillon
salt and freshly ground pepper
4 slices of rye or spelt bread,
  cut into cubes, to serve

Add the oil to a large pot, then add the shallot, garlic, and cardamom, and cook gently for 2–3 minutes. Stir in the leeks and bay leaves. Add the bouillon and bring to a boil. Turn down the heat and let simmer for 15 minutes. Season to taste with salt and freshly ground pepper.

Toast the bread cubes in a dry pan until golden brown, tossing them frequently and being careful not to let them burn.

Serve the soup very hot, scattered with the croutons.

TIP This is a very easy vegetable soup, and can be used with different vegetables; if you add potatoes and root vegetables, use 2¼ lbs peeled weight and then blend it when cooked and season to taste.

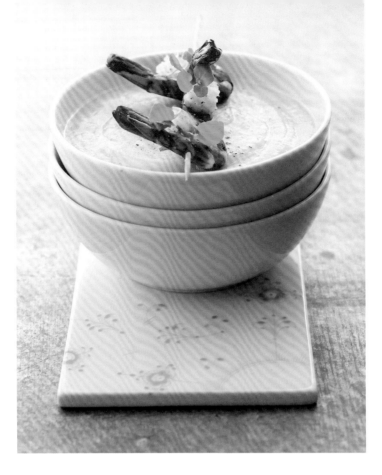

Cauliflower soup spiced with green chili and served with shrimp

People either love cauliflower or can't stand its funny, earthy taste. I love it and eat it raw, in a soup, or in curries. My grandmother would boil it for a long time, then serve it whole with shrimp around it and a white sauce on the side. This is my modern version of that recipe. Cauliflower is a good source of potassium, vitamin C, and folate, and it contains phytochemicals that fight many cancers. SERVES 4

1 large cauliflower
1 green chili, seeded and chopped
5 scallions, chopped
2 baking potatoes, peeled and cut
  into cubes
2 tsp salt and freshly ground pepper

to serve

14 oz shelled, cooked, extra-large
  cold water shrimp
watercress
spelt bread

Cut the cauliflower with the stalk into large pieces. Place all the ingredients in a large pan with 6⅓ cups of water. Cover with a lid and bring to a boil. Reduce the heat and let it simmer for 20 minutes.

With a hand blender, blend to a smooth soup and then reheat. Season to taste with salt and pepper.

Arrange the shrimp on 4 wooden skewers and serve them on top of the soup. Garnish with watercress sprigs and serve with spelt bread.

TIP This soup can also be made with broccoli.

Smørrebrød with salmon tartare

In Denmark smørrebrød *(open sandwiches) are eaten by lots of people every day for lunch—the permutations of healthy rye bread topped with fresh ingredients are endless. Nordic salmon, both marinated and cured, is world-famous, but serving it raw with horseradish is a great combination, providing lots of brain-boosting omega-3 fatty acids, protein, and minerals. For this treatment it is essential that you have a good supplier to ensure the salmon is very fresh.* SERVES 4

14 oz very fresh salmon fillet,
   skinned
2 cucumbers, halved and seeded
2 tbsp grated fresh horseradish
juice of 1 lime
1 tsp white wine vinegar
6 tbsp chopped chervil, plus
   4 sprigs to decorate
salt and freshly ground pepper
4 slices of rye bread
8 crisp lettuce leaves

Cut the salmon fillet into small squares and place in a bowl. Cut the cucumbers into cubes. Add to the salmon with the horseradish, lime juice, vinegar, and chopped chervil. Mix well and season with salt and pepper.

Place a slice of bread on each plate, place 2 lettuce leaves on each slice of bread, then spoon the salmon salad onto the lettuce leaves. Sprinkle with pepper and top with a sprig of chervil.

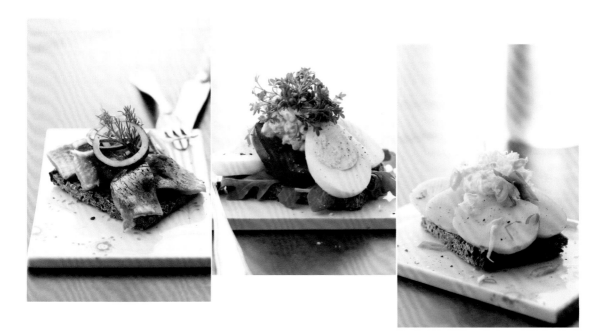

3 smørrebrød for everyday lunches

Rye is higher than wheat in fiber, vitamins B2, B5, and E, as well as folate. Unusual for a grain, it also contains twice as much of the amino acid lysine as wheat, so eating rye helps give you well-rounded protein in a low-meat diet. SERVES 2

Herring on rye bread

2 slices of rye bread
5 oz white herring in brine, or rollmops
20 slices of red onion
6 sprigs of dill
salt and freshly ground pepper

Place the bread slices on a small serving board or plate. Place the pieces of marinated herring on top of them, followed by the onion slices and the dill. Season and serve right away.

Egg and tomato on rye bread

2 tbsp cottage cheese
1 tsp Dijon mustard
salt and freshly ground pepper
2 slices of rye bread
¾ oz arugula leaves
2 organic hard-boiled eggs, sliced
2 tomatoes, sliced
cress

Mix the cottage cheese and mustard with some salt and pepper.

Place the bread slices on a small serving board or plate. Put some arugula leaves on them, followed by the egg and tomato slices. Spoon 1 tablespoon of the cottage cheese mixture on top and sprinkle with salt and pepper. Place the cress on top and serve right away.

Potatoes on rye bread

2 slices of rye bread
7 oz boiled new potatoes, sliced
1 tbsp chopped scallion

horseradish cream
2 tbsp Greek yogurt (10% fat)
1 tbsp shredded fresh horseradish, plus more to serve
½ tsp sugar
1 tbsp lemon juice
salt and freshly ground pepper

Make the horseradish cream by mixing all of the ingredients.

Place the bread slices on a small serving board or plate. Arrange the potato slices on them, place a tablespoon of the cream on top, and then sprinkle with scallion and salt and pepper. Place some horseradish on top of the cream. Serve right away.

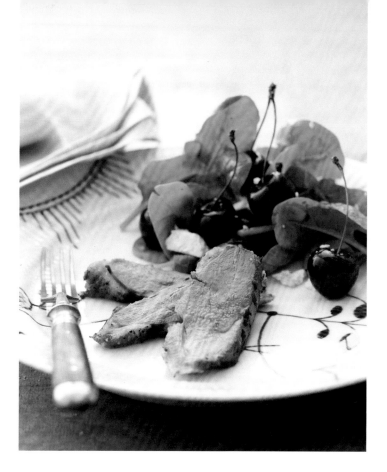

Spinach, duck breast, and cherry salad

In Scandinavia, cherries are in season in late July and August, and I eat a lot of these summer treats during the day. I also use them in salads and with other foods, both cold and hot. Cherries are rich in a phytochemical called ellagic acid that is thought to help fight cancer. SERVES 4

2 duck breasts
1 tsp coriander seeds
salt and freshly ground pepper
3½ oz baby spinach
1 tbsp grapeseed oil
7 oz cherries
2 tbsp raspberry vinegar
5 oz goat feta cheese, crumbled

Preheat the oven to 400°F. Cut the fat on top of the duck breast down to the flesh in a lattice pattern.

Crush the coriander seeds and rub the duck breast with them. Place in an ovenproof dish and sprinkle with salt and pepper. Cook in the oven for 20 minutes. Take out and let cool.

Rinse the spinach in cold water. Drain and set aside in a colander.

Heat the oil in a skillet and sauté the cherries for 3–5 minutes. Pour the vinegar over them, sprinkle with salt and pepper, and let cool down in the skillet.

Cut the duck breasts into thin slices. Spread the spinach leaves out on a large serving dish, then spread out the cherries and the feta on top of them. Sprinkle with salt and pepper, and mix the salad.

Serve the duck breast slices as an accompaniment to the salad or mixed in with it.

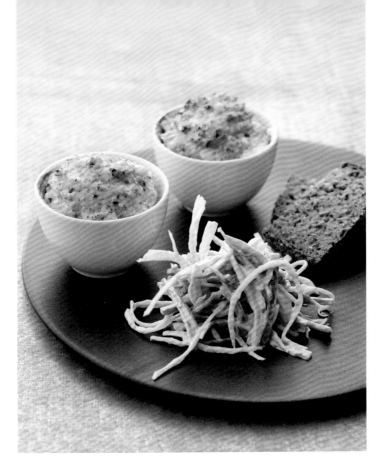

Baked fish with coleslaw

This is easy to do for weekend lunches, but save one for Monday's lunchbox. You can use cod or any white fish. SERVES 4–6

1 lb 2 oz skinless fillets of pollack
2 scallions, chopped
1 tbsp chopped lovage (or parsley, chervil, or dill)
whites of 2 eggs
generous ⅓ cup sparkling water
⅔ cup oats
salt and freshly ground pepper
a little butter for the cocottes
4 slices of rye bread, to serve

coleslaw

7 oz white cabbage
2 carrots, shredded
1 tbsp toasted sesame seeds

dressing

2 tbsp mustard powder
2 tbsp white wine vinegar
1 tsp honey
3 tbsp low-fat yogurt

Preheat the oven to 400°F.

Cut the fish fillets into smaller pieces, place into a food processor, and grind the fish meat (but not to a mush). Add the scallions and herbs. Blend for 1 minute, then add the egg whites and blend for 2 more minutes.

Take the mixture out of the food processor and place in a big mixing bowl. Add the sparkling water, oats, and salt and pepper to taste. Butter 4 or 6 cocottes and divide the fish mixture between them. Bake in the preheated oven for 15 minutes.

To make the coleslaw, mince the cabbage and mix with the carrot and sesame seeds. Mix together the dressing ingredients and then mix this in with the coleslaw. Season to taste with salt and pepper.

Serve the fish while still warm, with the coleslaw and rye bread.

TIP If you want to eat fishcakes instead, then just form the fish mixture into small burgers and cook in a little butter for 4–5 minutes, turning them once.

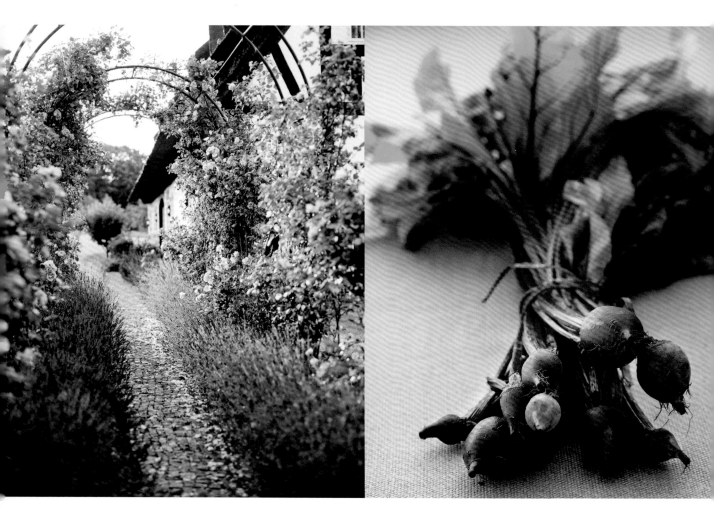

Beet contains moderate amounts of carbohydrates and is a good source of vitamin C and potassium, which together play a role in muscle contraction and thus the regulation of the heartbeat. It is also a useful source of bioflavonoids and carotenoids, antioxidants that help reduce oxidation of HDL (good) cholesterol, protecting artery walls and reducing the risk of heart disease and stroke. The natural sugars in the beet also aid the absorption of these potent phytochemicals. Beet is also one of the richest sources of folic acid, which helps protect unborn babies from spina bifida.

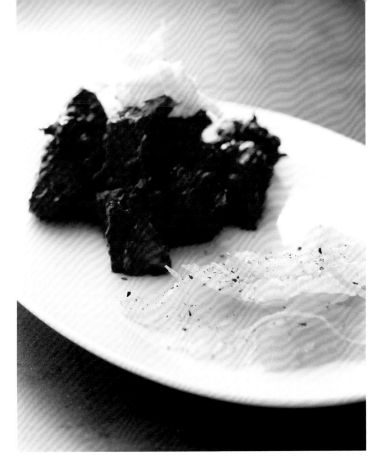

Salted pollack with beet salad

Eat fish as often as possible. A healthy and low-fat way to get your daily protein, it is also perfect for lunch as it is light and easy to digest. Pollack is a member of the cod family and is just as nutritious as cod although rather less flavorful. Low in saturated fat, it is a good source of riboflavin, niacin, vitamin B6, magnesium, and potassium, and a very good source of protein, vitamin B12, phosphorus, and the antioxidant mineral selenium. It also has the distinct advantage of not being as overfished a species as cod. SERVES 4

14 oz skinless pollack fillet
2 tbsp sea salt or another
  flaky salt
1 tsp sugar
grated zest from ½ of an unwaxed
  lemon
rye bread, to serve

beet salad
14 oz beet
4 tbsp grated fresh horseradish
2 tbsp lime juice
generous ¾ cup low-fat yogurt
salt and freshly ground pepper

Well ahead, place the fish in a big, deep oven tray with straight sides. Mix the salt, sugar, and lemon zest, then spread this mixture on both sides of the fish fillets. Cover the dish and leave it in the refrigerator for 4 hours.

To make the beet salad, first boil the beets in salted water for 30 minutes. Take out of the water and rinse in cold water, then peel and cut into ¾-inch cubes. Mix the beet with the horseradish, lime juice, and yogurt. Season to taste with salt and pepper.

When the fish has marinated for 4 hours, lightly brush the salt mixture off the fish, then cut the fillets into very thin slices.

Serve with the beet salad and rye bread.

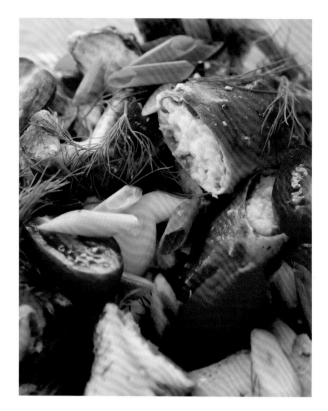

King crab salad

The giant Red King Crab is native to the Northern Pacific and Bering Sea. Biologists from the Soviet Union put the crab into European waters as an experiment, and at first the scientists thought the experiment was a failure until the king crabs starting showing up in large numbers in the 1970s, and now you can catch them further down the western part of the Norwegian coastline. Crabmeat is very rich in health-giving omega-3 fatty acids and is also a good source of the infection-fighting mineral zinc, which is otherwise quite difficult to come by in the average diet. SERVES 4

2¼ lbs king crab legs
2 large sprigs of dill, chopped
7 oz small plum tomatoes, cut in half
2 scallions, cut into thin slices
1 red chili, minced
juice from 1 lemon
2 tbsp extra virgin olive oil
salt and freshly ground pepper
spelt bread (page 138) or rye buns
 (page 130), to serve

brine

2 tbsp coarse sea salt
1 tbsp whole peppercorns
5 slices of unwaxed lemon

First make the brine: Pour 5¼ quarts of water into a large pot and add the salt, peppercorns, and lemon slices. Bring to a boil. Once boiling, add the king crab legs, cover, and let simmer for 7 minutes. At the end of this time, take out the crab legs and let them cool.

When they are cool, using a big, sharp kitchen knife, cut them into smaller pieces about ¾–1¼ inches, and place these in a big bowl. Add the dill, tomatoes, scallions, chili, lemon juice, and olive oil, and gently mix everything around. Season with salt and pepper and mix again.

Serve right away with spelt bread or rye buns.

TIP It is a good idea to serve the salad with lobster forks, so you can get all the juicy crabmeat out of the shells.

Nordic taramasalata with rye bread

This is my Nordic version of taramasalata, using cod's roe. If you can't get cod's roe, then you can use roe from other local fish in season. Although fish eggs, like hens' eggs, are high in cholesterol, they are an excellent source of vitamin C, thiamin, and folate, and a very good source of protein, vitamin E, riboflavin, vitamin B12, phosphorus, and selenium, so high in protective antioxidants. They are also high in omega-3 fatty acids. SERVES 4 (OR 2 FOR LUNCH FOR 2 DAYS)

14 oz cod's roe
1 scallion, chopped
2 tbsp each chopped dill and chives
2 tbsp extra virgin canola or olive oil
3 tbsp lemon juice or to taste

brine
1 tbsp coarse sea salt
1 tbsp whole black peppercorns
3 slices of lemon

First make the brine: Pour scant 3¼ quarts of water into a large pot and add the brine ingredients. Bring to a boil, place the roe in the brine, and simmer for 30 minutes. Take the roe out of the water with a slotted spoon and let cool.

Remove and discard the membrane from the roe, place in a food processor with the other ingredients, and blend until you have an even paste. Take out of the food processor and season with salt and pepper.

Serve with rye toast and a green salad, dressed with a little lemon juice. TIP If you make a portion and store it in the refrigerator for your lunchbox, it will last for three days.

Salads

Salads are also a very good means of eating all kinds of vegetables—and fruit. Mixed salads can also be very important parts of a balanced diet, as they provide you with a broad range of different healthy foods each with its own mixture of nutrients. You also are assured of getting the best of the goodness in the ingredients as you are generally enjoying them raw. Salads are also a great challenge for the cook's imagination—don't hesitate to try your own combinations.

Green salad with radish, smoked mackerel and smoked herring

In summer I serve this salad for either dinner or lunch, as it is both filling and fresh, making the perfect light meal on a hot day. SERVES 4

7 oz smoked mackerel or herring
14 oz boiled new potatoes, sliced
3½ oz frisée leaves, torn into pieces
3½ oz corn salad
10 radishes, sliced
4 tbsp chopped chives
5 oz small tomatoes, halved
rye bread, to serve

dressing
⅔ cup low-fat plain yogurt
2 tbsp Dijon mustard
2 tbsp lemon juice
salt and freshly ground pepper

Remove the skin and any bones from the smoked fish and divide the flesh into smaller pieces. Mix these and all the remaining salad ingredients in a serving bowl.

Make the dressing by mixing all the ingredients together. Serve the salad with rye bread and the dressing on the side.

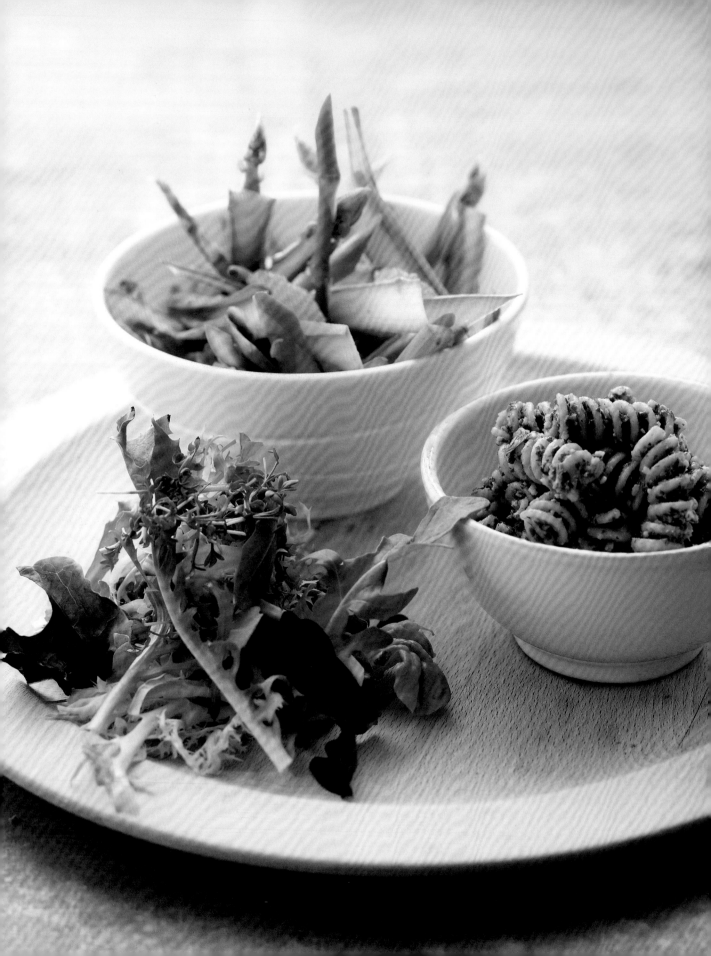

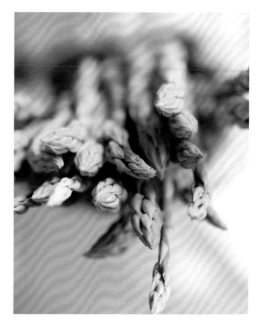

ASPARAGUS. When I was a child we had asparagus only once every spring and it was a real luxury, like lobster. I only liked the fresh green stalks and never liked white asparagus from a can, which I found slimy and too sweet. It took me years to realize that the canned item could have anything to do with the green stalks I tasted each May, because I didn't come across the white blanched stalks so popular in Spain until I was in my twenties. Asparagus is considered a "superfood" by many, as it is one of the few vegetable sources of vitamin E. The glucosides it contains are thought to be anti-inflammatory and useful in easing rheumatoid arthritis.

Spring salads

Serve these two salads together with a simple green salad for supper with home-baked bread. SERVES 4

Asparagus salad

1 bunch of asparagus
2 lemons
2 tbsp pine nuts
1 tbsp virgin olive oil
salt and freshly ground pepper

Break off the lowest third of each asparagus stalk (save the ends for a vegetable stock or soup) and cut the stalks lengthwise into very thin slices.

Peel one whole lemon, removing all the bitter white pith under the skin. Cut out each segment of lemon flesh by cutting down in between the membranes and the flesh.

Toast the pine nuts in a dry pan until golden (this takes a couple of minutes and be careful not to let them burn).

Mix the asparagus, lemon segments, and pine nuts together in a mixing bowl with the juice of the second lemon and the olive oil. Season to taste with salt and pepper.

Spring spelt pasta salad with ground-elder pesto

11 oz spelt pasta

ground-elder pesto
3½ oz ground-elder, top leaves only
1 small garlic clove, chopped
3 tbsp extra virgin canola oil or olive oil
¼ cup almonds
3 tbsp lemon juice
salt and freshly ground pepper

GROUND-ELDER (Aegopodium podagraria) is a member of the carrot family that generally grows in shady places. Also known as goutweed, goatweed, and snow-in-the-mountain, it is said to have been introduced to Britain as a food plant by the Romans and then to Northern Europe by monks in the Middle Ages, who cultivated it as a healing herb. Culpeper noted that "it is found to heal the gout (hence the alternative name) and sciatica. It is also used for aching joints and other cold pains." It is a common pest in shrubbery and ill-kept gardens, and it is found on the outskirts of almost every village or town. In spring, garden lovers spend a lot of time digging up the plants and disposing of them, but why not pick the top leaves in spring and use them in pestos or salads as you would spinach.

Pick the ground-elder fresh in spring only, then rinse in cold water and drain in a colander. Place in a food processor with the other ingredients except the salt and pepper, and blend to a smooth paste. Season to taste with salt and pepper and perhaps more lemon juice.

Boil the spelt pasta in lightly salted water for 8–10 minutes until al dente. Drain in a colander and let it cool down. When cool, place in a mixing bowl, mix with the pesto, and season again with salt and pepper.
TIP If you don't have the opportunity of picking ground-elder, then use parsley, arugula, or dandelion leaves (the dandelion only in spring).

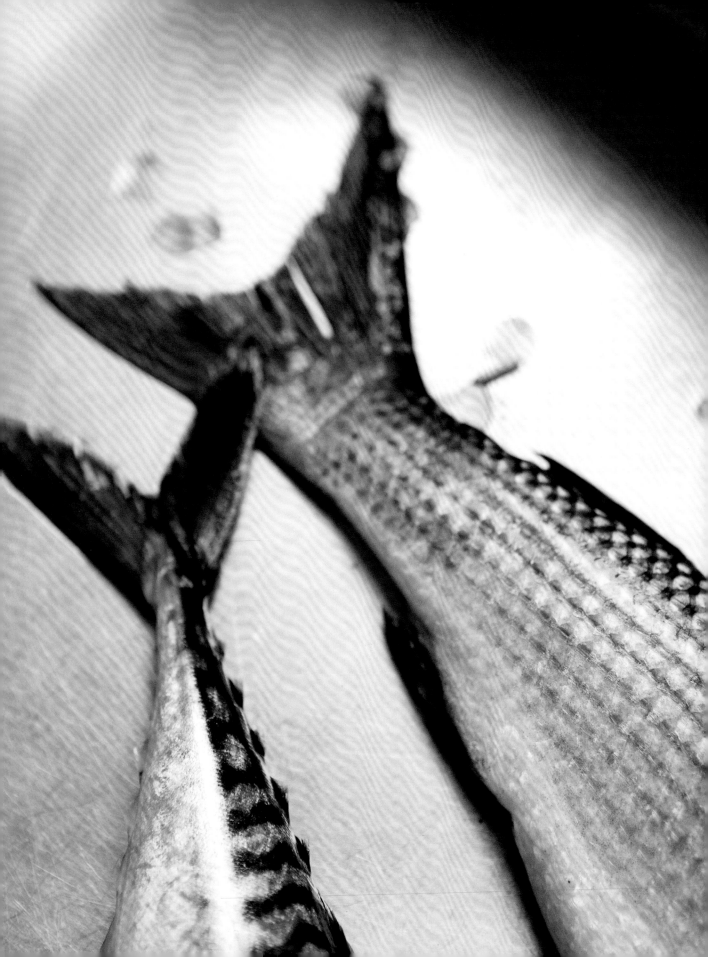

Smoked mackerel salad on rye bread

Smoked mackerel is best in August as the mackerel has by then become fully grown and is therefore a bit fattier, which makes it perfect to smoke. It can also be quite overpowering in its taste in August if just pan-fried. Mackerel is one of the richest sources of omega-3 fatty acids, which are vital for good heart and brain health, helping to make the blood less sticky. SERVES 2

½ smoked mackerel
½ cucumber, thinly sliced
1 small red onion, minced
1 bunch of chives, minced
1 tbsp capers, rinsed and drained
1 hard-boiled egg, minced
3½ oz frisée leaves
salt and freshly ground pepper

to serve
2 slices of rye bread
5–6 radishes, chopped

Carefully remove and discard all bones and skin from the mackerel and break up the mackerel meat into small pieces.

Mix the mackerel, cucumber, onion, chives, capers, egg, and frisée leaves in a bowl. Season to taste with salt and pepper.

Serve the mixture on rye bread, topped with chopped radishes.

RADISHES are among the oldest cultivated plants we have. They originate from China, and the Egyptians grew radishes before the time of the pyramids. They are extremely easy to grow, developing in a very short time, and can therefore be sown several times during spring, summer, and early fall. They have a high content of folate, vitamin C, potassium, and mustard oil, which has antibacterial properties.

Summer salads

That you can't get full on vegetables alone is a myth—it is just another kind of feeling where you can still move and don't have to lie down for half an hour after dinner to let your food be digested. What I want to emphasize is that you might need to get used to not eating meat every day; changing your diet from meat to a lot of vegetables will give you energy after meals, but it can take a few weeks to adjust. However, you will certainly soon feel the benefits. SERVES 4

Pointed cabbage with shrimp, watercress, and radish

5½ oz pointed cabbage
7 oz cooked and peeled cold water shrimp
5 oz radishes, sliced
2 oz watercress
2 tbsp white wine vinegar
1 tbsp extra virgin canola oil or virgin olive oil
salt and freshly ground pepper

Cut the cabbage into slices, rinse in cold water, and drain in a colander.

In a mixing bowl, mix the cabbage, shrimp, radishes, watercress, vinegar, and oil. Season to taste with salt and pepper. Serve right away.

Tomato and cucumber salad with fresh mint

1 cucumber
9 oz red and yellow cherry tomatoes (or big ones)
2 tbsp chopped mint
salt and freshly ground pepper
juice from ½ lemon

Cut the cucumber in half lengthwise and scrape out the seeds, then cut in slices. Cut the tomatoes in half.

In a serving bowl, mix the cucumber, tomatoes, mint, and lemon juice. Season to taste with salt and pepper, and serve.

Fennel salad with strawberries, goat feta, and raspberry vinaigrette

1 head of fennel
1 cup strawberries
1 cup crumbled goat feta

dressing
½ cup raspberries
2 tbsp raspberry vinegar

Cut the fennel in super-thin slices on a mandoline grater, then place the slices in a bowl of cold water so they will curl up. Leave for half an hour. Take them out of the water and drain in a colander.

Cut the strawberries into slices and mix with the fennel and the goat feta.

Make the dressing: Add the raspberries and raspberry vinegar to a blender and blend until well mixed. Arrange the salad on a serving platter, dribble the dressing over it, and serve right away.

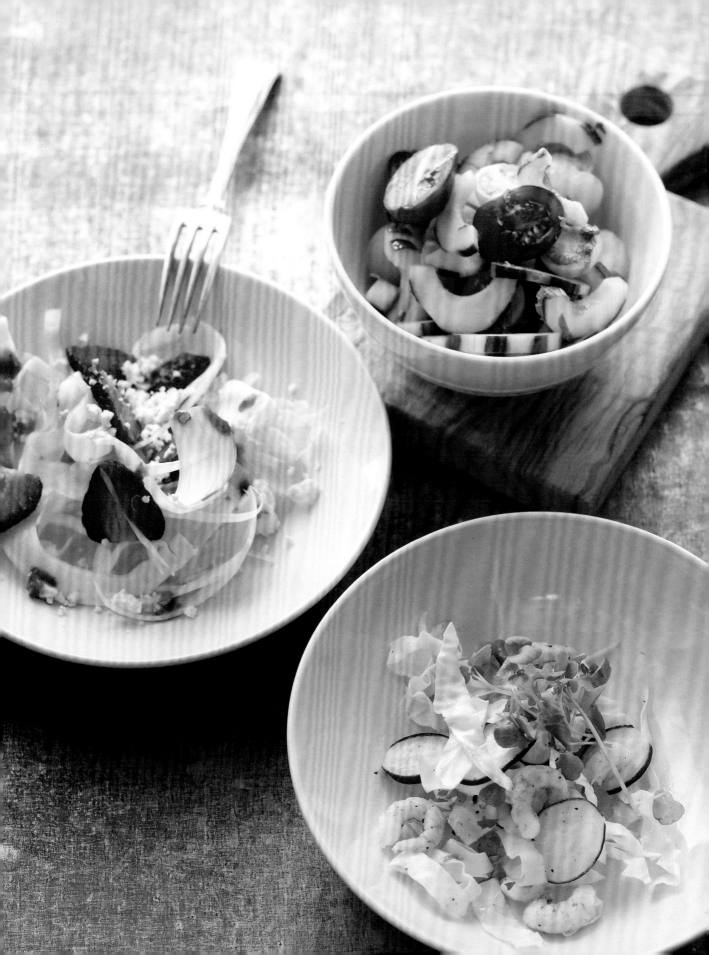

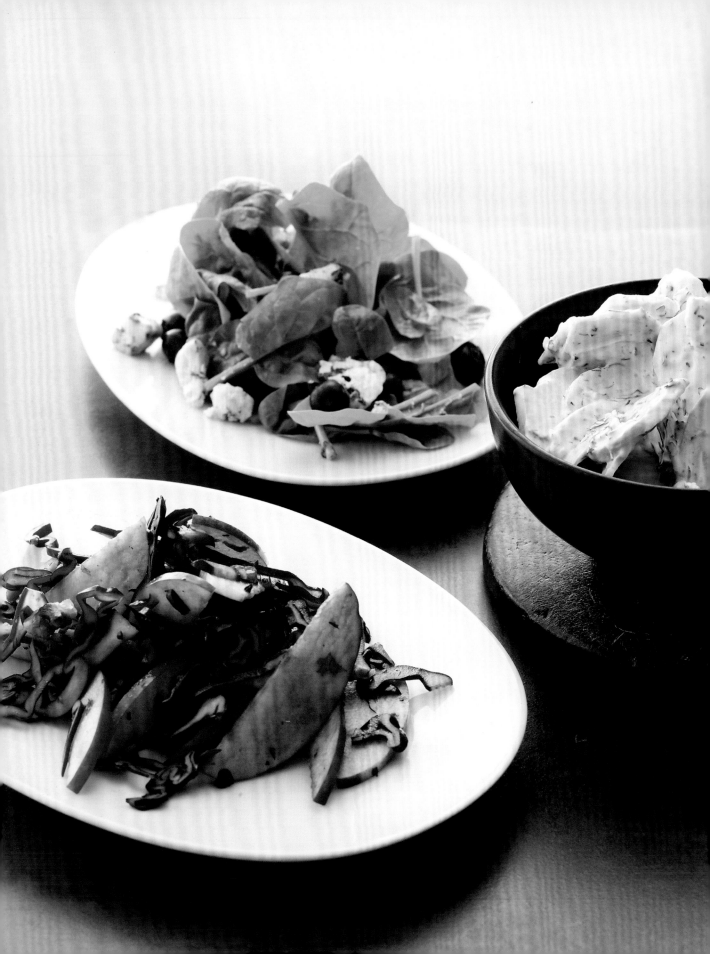

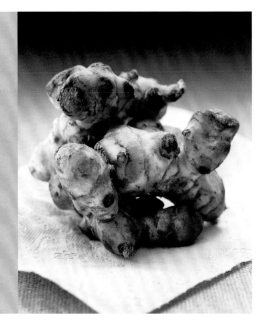

JERUSALEM ARTICHOKES, originally cultivated by Native Americans, are very low in saturated fat, cholesterol, and sodium but rich in iron and a good source of antioxidant vitamin C, as well as thiamin, phosphorus, and potassium. They also contain a good deal of probiotics, i.e., nondigestible food ingredients that stimulate healthy bacteria growth in the human digestive system. The plant is extremely easy to grow and the yield astonishing. The season starts in October. You then can dig them all up, but as they can be difficult to store it is best to keep them in the earth during the winter. They can be harvested until March/April.

Fall salads

In the fall there are all the root vegetables, which you can use for a lot of different salads. Basically they can all be baked and served with a yogurt or oil and vinegar dressing, while beet, carrots, and Jerusalem artichokes can also be eaten raw, although the latter need to be thinly sliced or grated. Serve all three of the following salads together for supper, with home-baked spelt bread, or serve them separately to accompany meat or fish. SERVES 4

Jerusalem artichoke salad with cold sauce verte

1¼ lbs Jerusalem artichokes

sauce verte
generous ⅓ cup low-fat yogurt
2 tbsp chopped dill
2 tbsp chopped parsley
1 tsp lemon juice
salt and freshly ground pepper

Mix all the ingredients for the sauce verte in a large mixing bowl.

Peel the Jerusalem artichokes and cut into very thin slices, adding them directly to the sauce verte to make sure they do not discolor. Season to taste with salt and pepper.

Salad with blueberries and blue cheese

5 oz fresh spinach leaves
1 cup blueberries or any berry or fruit in season
3 oz blue cheese, cut into small cubes

dressing
2 tbsp balsamic vinegar
1 tbsp canola oil or olive oil
salt and freshly ground pepper

Rinse the spinach in plenty of cold water three or four times. Drain in a colander. Rinse the blueberries and drain well.

Place the spinach in a big bowl and mix in the blueberries and blue cheese. Whisk the dressing ingredients together and mix in with the salad. Season to taste with salt and pepper.

Raw red cabbage salad

½ cup walnuts
7 oz red cabbage, finely shredded
1 apple, thinly sliced

dressing
1 tsp apple jelly
1½ tbsp white wine vinegar
1 tbsp walnut oil
salt and freshly ground pepper

Toast the walnuts carefully in a dry pan until golden, then chop them roughly.

Mix the red cabbage, apples, and walnuts in a serving bowl.

Make the dressing by whisking together the apple jelly and vinegar, then whisk in the oil. Season to taste with salt and pepper. Mix into the cabbage salad and serve.

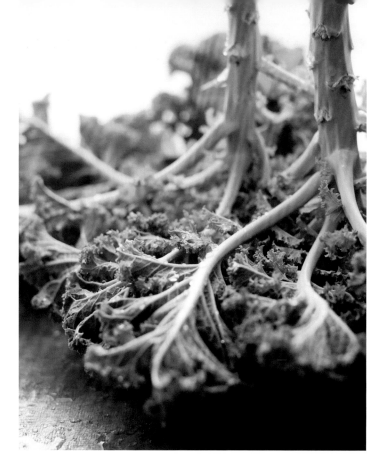

Kale and chicken salad

Kale is a winter superfood; use it for salad in place of lettuce, in pasta dishes, and add to mashed potatoes—think of your own ways to use kale in your everyday winter food. SERVES 4

1 organic chicken
1 tbsp salt
1 tbsp whole peppercorns
2 bay leaves
11 oz celeriac
11 oz raw kale
spelt bread (page 138), to serve

dressing
1 tbsp Dijon mustard
3 tbsp lemon juice
1 tbsp extra virgin olive oil
1 tbsp chopped capers

Gently boil the chicken in scant 3¼ quarts of water with the salt, peppercorns, and bay leaves for an hour. Let cool in the stock.

Preheat the oven to 400°F. Peel the celeriac and cut it into sticks. Place these in an ovenproof dish and sprinkle with salt and pepper. Bake in the preheated oven for 20 minutes and allow these to cool down as well.

Take the chicken out of the stock and save the stock for soup or risotto. Skin the chicken and remove the flesh from the bones.

Mince the kale and mix with the chicken and celeriac in a serving bowl.

Make the dressing by mixing the mustard and lemon juice, then slowly add the oil and the capers. Mix into the salad and season to taste with salt and pepper.

Serve with spelt bread.

Kale is a fantastic source of soluble fiber, the antioxidant vitamins A, C, and K, and the energy-releasing B vitamins, as well as large amounts of sulfur-containing phytochemicals now known to protect against some cancers. It is also a good natural source of folate for pregnant women, and lutein, a phytochemical with powerful antioxidant properties important for maintaining healthy vision. Kale is easy to grow, particularly in colder temperatures, where a light frost will produce especially sweet leaves.

Winter salads

You can make tasty salads all year round; simply combine winter vegetables in all kinds of ways, and mix them with different dressings. Serve the following three salads together as supper with a spelt baguette (page 137). SERVES 4

Potato and kale salad

Winter potatoes are not very tasty and often very mushy, and are therefore best roasted, mashed, or dressed in a salad.

14 oz potatoes
1 lb 2 oz raw kale

dressing
2 tbsp grainy mustard
2 tbsp hot mustard
1 tsp honey
1 tbsp white wine vinegar
2 tbsp extra virgin canola oil or
   olive oil
salt and freshly ground pepper

Peel the potatoes if necessary, boil them until just tender, and then cut them into chunks. Cut away the stalks from the kale and then mince the leaves and mix with the potatoes.

Make the dressing by whisking the mustards, honey, and vinegar together and, still whisking, gradually add the oil. Season to taste with salt and pepper. Mix the dressing into the salad. Season again.

TIP This salad is very good with roast chicken or baked cod.

Brussels sprouts with apples and walnut oil

Remember never to overcook Brussels sprouts, as they then lose their fresh, green, nutty flavor and their crisp texture.

1 lb 2 oz Brussels sprouts
salt and freshly ground pepper
7 oz apples, sliced
1 green chili, seeded and
   chopped
2 tbsp apple cider vinegar
2 tbsp walnut oil

If necessary discard the outer leaves of the sprouts, then cut the sprouts in half. Cook them in salted boiling water for 5 minutes, then drain them.

In a serving bowl, mix the sprouts with the apple slices, chili, vinegar, and walnut oil, then season to taste with salt and pepper.

Salsify with red onion and parsley

Black salsify roots, also known as scorzonera, are usually very dirty and rather difficult to clean, but their flavor makes the work worthwhile.

1 lb 2 oz salsify
milk, to soak
1 tbsp canola oil
1 red onion, halved and sliced
salt and freshly ground pepper
8 tbsp roughly chopped Italian
   parsley

Peel the salsify and rinse in water, then cut into thick slices and put to soak in milk to prevent discoloration.

Pan-fry the drained slices in the oil in a skillet with the red onion for 3–5 minutes. Sprinkle with salt and pepper, transfer to a serving plate, and sprinkle with the parsley.

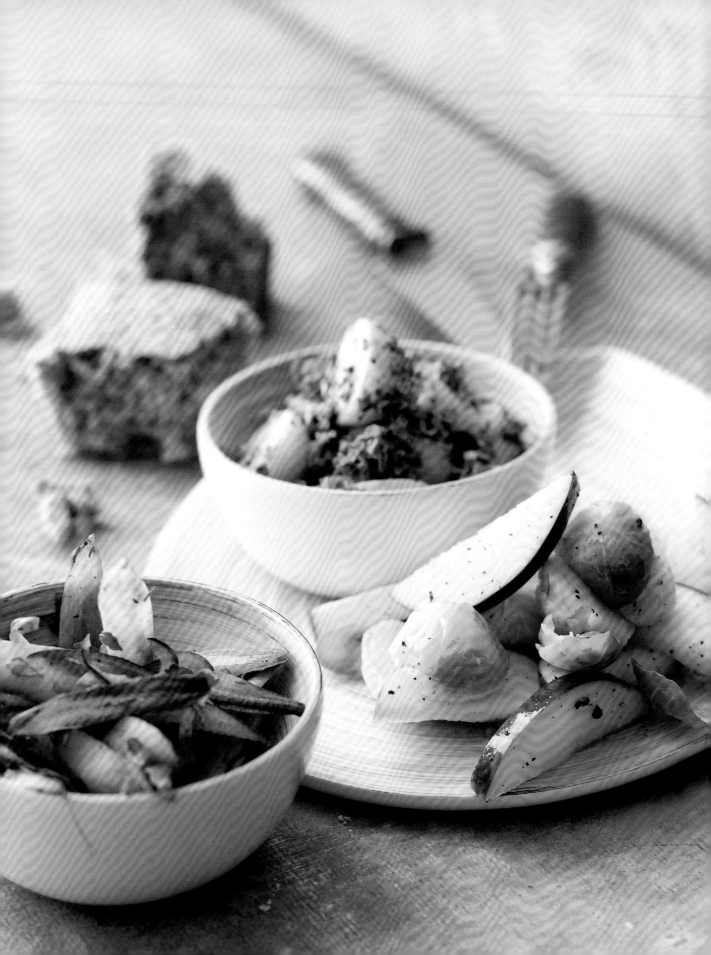

Vegetarian

The old concept of a meal always having to consist of "meat and two vegetables" is now well and truly buried. There is no nutritional requirement for us to eat meat or fish every day, as most of us actually get too much protein. For a healthy, balanced diet it is a good idea to have one or more vegetarian meals during the week, as they are full of fiber and all sorts of nutritional goodies. There are many days during the week where I prepare a nice big salad, a vegetarian stew, or pasta with vegetables. The important thing is that it has to be gastronomically interesting; it has to contain lots of flavors and texture. So use your imagination and experiment with all the wonderful array of vegetables, herbs, and spices.

Mashed potato with a mixed vegetable topping

This mash with sautéed leeks, celery, beet, and walnuts is actually quite easy to prepare and makes a very tasty vegetarian dinner. It is one of my winter favorites. SERVES 4

14 oz celeriac, peeled and cut
  into cubes
14 oz potatoes, peeled and cut
  into large cubes
2 garlic cloves, chopped
1 tsp whole peppercorns
1 tbsp sea salt flakes
2 bay leaves
2 tbsp canola oil or olive oil

mixed vegetable topping
1 tbsp canola oil
1 garlic clove, chopped
7 oz raw beet, peeled and
  cut into very small cubes
2 celery stalks, minced
2 leeks, minced
½ cup walnuts, chopped
salt and freshly ground pepper

To a large pot add the celeriac, potatoes, garlic, peppercorns, salt, and bay leaves. Cover generously with water, bring to a boil, and then let simmer for 30 minutes.

While the vegetables are cooking, prepare the topping: Heat the oil in a sauté pan, add the garlic and beet, and cook gently for 5 minutes. Add the rest of the vegetables and the walnuts. Continue cooking for 5 minutes more. Season to taste with salt and pepper. Keep the sauce warm.

Drain the vegetables and place in a big bowl, discarding the bay leaves. Add the canola or olive oil and mash, mixing everything well together. Season to taste with salt and pepper.

Serve the mash in a large bowl, topped with the mixed vegetables.

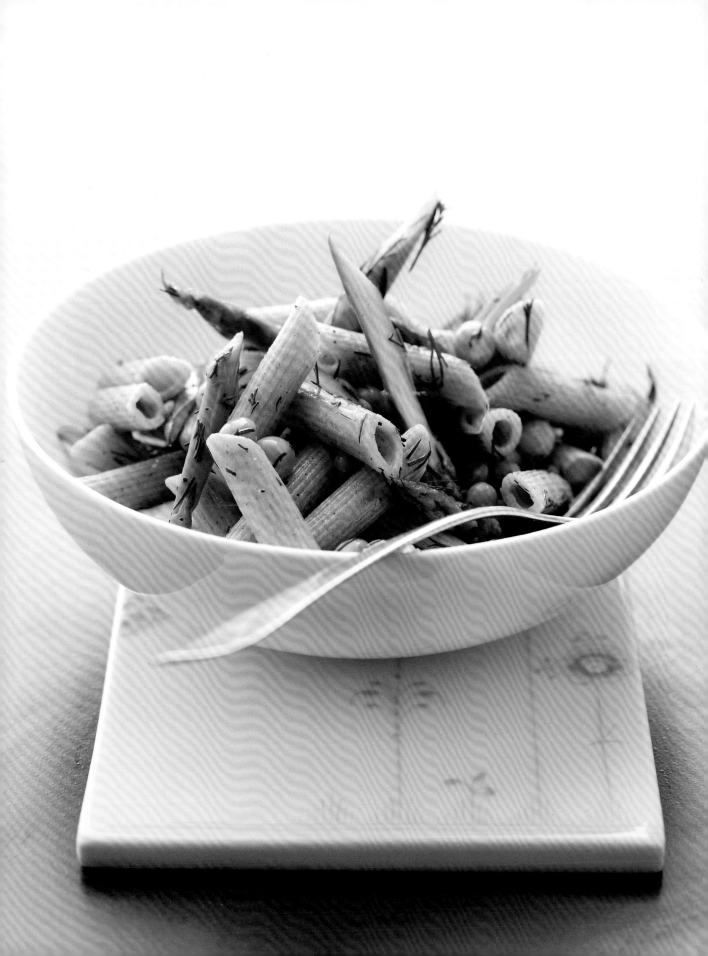

DILL is an ancient medical herb even mentioned in the Bible. It is rich in niacin, phosphorus, zinc, and copper, and it is a very good source of vitamins A and C, riboflavin, vitamin B6, folate, calcium, iron, magnesium, potassium, and manganese. It also contains cancer-fighting phytochemicals and is antibacterial. Cooking ruins the taste, so always add it at the very last minute. It is very easy to grow, often self-sowing. The season is from June to late fall.

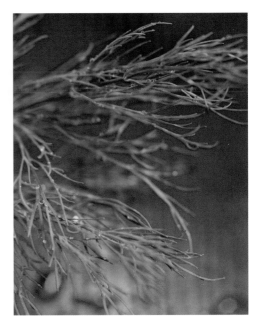

Spelt pasta with scallions, asparagus, dill, and peas

If you don't have much time to cook every day, it is a very healthy and easy solution to prepare pasta dishes with lots of vegetables and serve them with a green salad. I also believe that it is a myth that we should not have pasta for dietary reasons. We can, of course, not eat pasta portions the size of Mount Everest, but dishes with 3–3½ oz of pasta per person, depending on body weight, are fine. Remember that the planet's population grew to over 6 billion people mainly on wheat and rice. Pasta also contains protein and the level of protein is even higher in spelt pasta. SERVES 4

1 bunch of asparagus
14 oz spelt pasta
salt and freshly ground pepper
1–2 tbsp olive oil
1 garlic clove, chopped
3 scallions, cut into pieces
2 cups peas, shelled weight
4 tbsp chopped dill

Break off and discard the lowest third of the asparagus where it snaps naturally and cut the remaining stalk in half lengthwise.

Cook the pasta in salted boiling water, not stirring for the first 3 minutes as spelt pasta breaks easily, until al dente, about 8–10 minutes.

While the pasta is cooking, heat the olive oil in a sauté pan and add the garlic, asparagus, scallions, and peas. Cook gently for 5 minutes over medium heat. Take care that the garlic does not burn.

Drain the cooked pasta; mix with the vegetables and season to taste with salt and pepper.

Serve right away, scattered with the dill.

TIP Here in the Nordic countries, we also eat our pasta with Parmesan or Grana Padano. I really love my vegetable pasta with a scattering of nice cheese on top. I really believe we should nurture inspirations we have received from other food cultures and I will never give up what I have learned from my European neighbors. We cannot—and should not—roll back time.

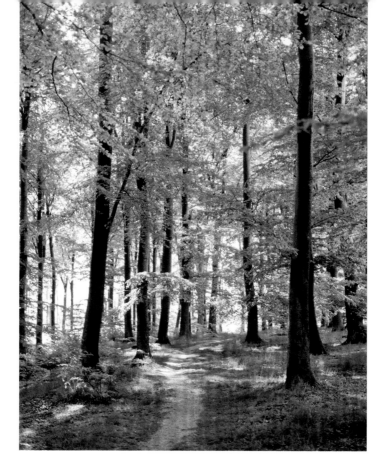

Brown rice risotto with mushrooms

Mushrooms are the pearls of fall and the perfect match for risotto or pasta dishes, and this risotto is a very filling and tasty meal. I use the mushrooms that I can get, but my favorites are the chanterelles and Karl Johan (our name for cep porcini) freshly picked from the Nordic woods. You really need to find the Italian brown risotto rice called "riso integrale" for this risotto. Ordinary brown rice won't give the same results. Brown rice is incredibly nutritious, "the perfect complex carbohydrate," packed full of B vitamins and the minerals selenium, manganese, magnesium, phosphorus, and copper, plus omega-3 fatty acids. SERVES 4 ·

scant 1¼ cups Italian risotto *riso integrale*
  (brown risotto rice)
1 tsp salt
11 oz mixed mushrooms
2 tbsp extra virgin olive oil
1 garlic clove, chopped
3 parsley stalks, minced and
  8 tbsp chopped parsley leaves
1¼ cups hot water
salt and freshly ground pepper

Rinse the rice thoroughly in cold water, then place it in a pan, and add enough fresh water to cover by ¾ inches above the top of the rice. Add the salt. Bring to a boil and let boil for 5 minutes. Drain and set aside.

Clean the mushrooms with a brush or your fingers, using as little water as possible, and cut them roughly into smaller pieces.

Heat the oil in a sauté pan and sauté the garlic, mushrooms, and parsley stalks for 2 minutes, then add the rice and sauté for 5 minutes over medium heat.

Add the hot water, bring to a boil, and let simmer for 10 minutes, stirring now and then. Season to taste with salt and pepper. Mix in the chopped parsley and serve right away.

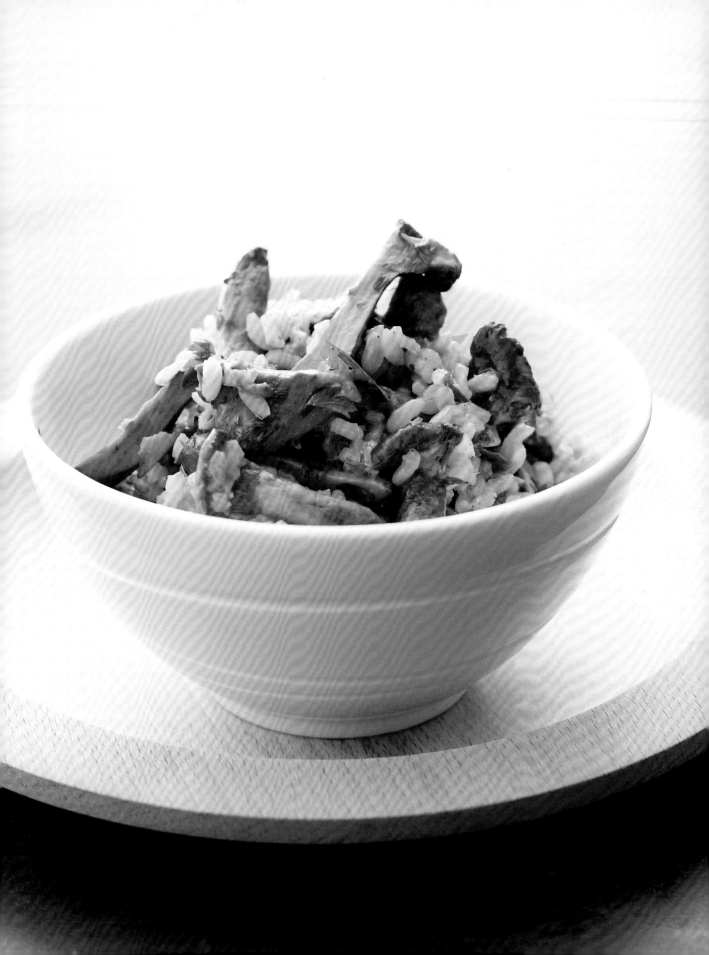

Rye pasta with kale and garlic

Nowadays, rye or spelt pasta can be very good quality. With kale, it makes a simple dish that is perfect during the week. As an additional bonus, it takes only 20 minutes to cook for dinner. SERVES 4

14 oz rye pasta
salt and freshly ground pepper
1 lb 2 oz fresh kale
2 tbsp virgin olive oil
2 garlic cloves, minced
1 fresh green chili, minced
side salad, to serve

Cook the pasta in salted boiling water, not stirring for the first 3 minutes as rye pasta breaks easily, until al dente, about 8–10 minutes.

Cut off and discard the tough stalks from the kale, roughly chop the leaves, and rinse well.

Heat the olive oil in a sauté pan, add the garlic and chili, and cook gently for 2 minutes.

Add the kale and continue to cook for 5 minutes. Season to taste with salt and pepper.

Drain the cooked pasta and mix the kale mixture into it. Serve right away with a side salad.

TIP In summer, replace the kale with broccoli.

Garlic originates from Southwest and Central Asia, and is now widely cultivated in southern and eastern Europe, and the Americas. The Ancient Greeks and the Romans regarded garlic as a curative and aphrodisiac. **It contains antioxidant vitamin C and B6, plus calcium and iron.** When garlic is chopped or crushed, it yields a compound called allicin, which is a potent antibacterial and antifungal. Garlic is easy to grow, even in cold climates. The best planting time is in October; then the bulbs can be harvested the following summer.

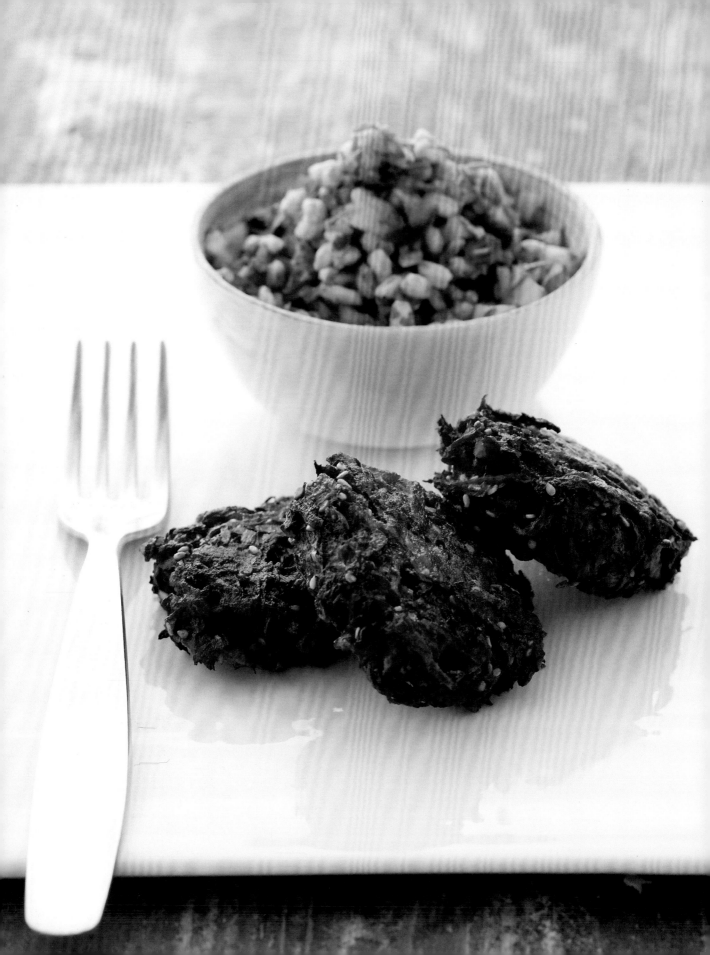

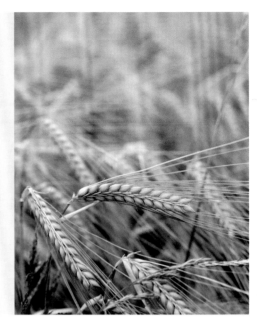

BARLEY was possibly the earliest grain crop that man cultivated and it is still one of the most widely grown grains all over the world, as it seems to thrive in a wide variety of soil types. Most of the crop, however, goes into animal feed and the brewing of beer. Scotch or pot barley, the complete grain, is rich in soluble dietary fiber, so helps lower blood cholesterol levels. It is rich in minerals, especially iron, manganese, potassium, selenium, and phosphorus, as well as some B vitamins. It also contains twice as much essential fatty acids as wheat.

Beet "burgers" with barley salad

Beet is in season from May to November, but tends to be smaller in the spring, and the fall harvest keeps well through the winter. A good rule is to go for the smaller ones for tenderness, especially if planning to use them raw in salads, and avoid very large ones, which may have a woody core. Try to get them with their leaves, which are also highly nutritious. SERVES 4

beet burgers
9 oz raw red beet, grated
9 oz raw yellow beet, grated
scant 1 cup oatmeal
3 eggs
1 shallot, minced
4 tbsp minced dill
2 tbsp minced thyme
2 tbsp minced parsley
salt and freshly ground pepper
1 tbsp canola oil, for pan-frying

barley salad
scant 1 cup barley
1 celery stalk, minced
1 big bunch of Italian parsley
1 tbsp extra virgin canola oil
   or olive oil
2 tbsp red wine vinegar

Mix the ingredients for the burgers well in a bowl, and let rest in the refrigerator for 1 hour.

Prepare the barley for the salad: Boil it in water with a little salt for 30 minutes. Drain and let cool down. Set aside.

Preheat the oven to 350°F. Form flat cakes of the burger mixture with your hands. Heat the oil in a skillet and pan-fry the cakes until golden on both sides. Transfer them to an ovenproof dish and put in the oven for 20 minutes.

Make the salad: Mix the barley with the celery, parsley, oil, and red wine vinegar. Season to taste with salt and pepper.

Serve the beet cakes with the barley salad. It is also a great idea to serve the horseradish sauce on page 91 with this dish.

TIP The burgers can be made the day before and reheated.

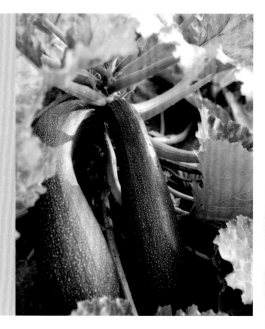

ZUCCHINI, *a type of summer squash, is one of the easiest vegetables to cultivate in temperate climates. There are several varieties in different colors and shapes; greens and yellows are the most familiar. The season is from June to early October. Some types, called winter zucchini, can be stored for months. The long green and yellow ones must be picked when under 8 inches in length or they become fibrous and inedible. Zucchini flowers are also very delicious and often stuffed with meat or cheese. Zucchini are low in calories and contain useful amounts of folate, vitamins A, C, and K, and several B vitamins, as well as a range of minerals, including phosphorus, copper, magnesium, and manganese.*

Basic rye pizza dough

Pizza is many things to many people, but basically it is a piece of flatbread with a topping that you eat warm. In the Nordic countries we have something similar, so this is my Nordic pizza. MAKES 2 (14-INCH) PIZZAS

1 oz yeast
1¼ cups lukewarm water
3 cups rye flour
scant 1 cup Italian tipo 00 flour or
  all-purpose flour
1 tsp salt

Dissolve the yeast in ¼ cup of the water, then add to a bowl containing a mixture of 2 tablespoons of the rye flour and 1 tablespoon Italian tipo 00 or all-purpose flour. Stir to a paste, then let rest, covered with a towel, for 30 minutes.

After the 30 minutes, stir in the remaining 1 cup lukewarm water and add the rest of the flour and the salt. Mix to a dough, then knead well until smooth. Place in a big bowl, cover with a towel, and let rise for 2 hours.

Rye pizza with potatoes
2 PIZZAS SERVES 4

1 portion of rye pizza dough
1½ tbsp olive oil

topping
1¾ lbs potatoes, cut into very thin slices
5 sprigs of rosemary, stems removed
salt and freshly ground pepper

Preheat the oven to 425°F. Roll the dough out to two very thin, large squares, each about 14 inches. Place on an oiled cookie sheet, then brush the tops with olive oil.

Place the potato slices evenly over the pizza dough, brush again with olive oil, scatter the rosemary on the top of the potato, and sprinkle with salt and pepper.

Bake for 20–25 minutes. Serve with a green salad.

Rye pizza with zucchini and tomato
2 PIZZAS SERVES 4

1 portion rye pizza dough
1½ tbsp olive oil

topping
2 zucchini, each about 9 oz, sliced
1 lb 2 oz small plum tomatoes, halved
9 oz buffalo mozzarella, torn into small pieces
scant 1 cup ricotta cheese
salt and freshly ground pepper

Preheat the oven to 425°F. Roll the dough out to 2 very thin, large squares, about 14 inches. Place on a lightly oiled cookie sheet, then brush the tops with olive oil.

Space the zucchini slices and tomato halves evenly out on the dough, then spread out the mozzarella and ricotta. Sprinkle with salt and pepper.

Bake for 20–25 minutes. Serve with a green salad.

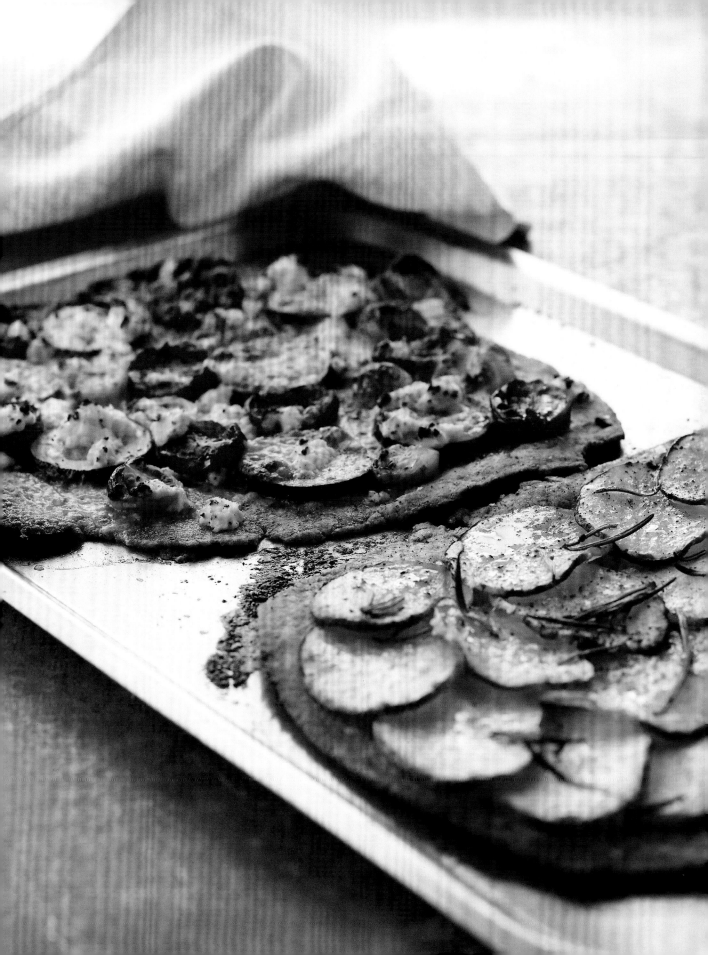

Vegetable biksemad with poached egg

This is my version of biksemad, *a traditional dish normally made using leftover meat and potatoes with onion and Worcestershire sauce. It is usually served with eggs fried sunny side up and tomato ketchup. I developed this recipe when I was a vegetarian for some years. Enjoy my* biksemad—*it is the best healthy hangover food in the world.* SERVES 4

2 tbsp olive oil
1 onion, chopped
7 oz peeled cooked beet,
  cut into cubes
1 ¼ lbs cold boiled potatoes,
  cut into cubes
2 carrots, cut into cubes
2 celery stalks, roughly chopped
salt and freshly ground pepper
4 large eggs (as fresh as possible)
about 6 tbsp vinegar
4 tbsp minced chives, to serve

Heat the oil in a skillet, then add the onion and beet. Cook gently over medium heat for 5 minutes, then add the potatoes and carrots and continue cooking for 10 more minutes. Lastly add the celery with some salt and pepper, and cook for 5 minutes more, stirring often so the vegetables do not stick to the pan.

Poach the eggs just before serving: Use a sauté pan deep enough to hold 2¾–3¼ inches of water and big enough to accommodate all 4 eggs at once. Add the vinegar (3 tablespoons per 4 cups of water) to the water and bring to a boil. Break each egg into a heatproof cup and carefully lower it into the water. Lower the heat and simmer for 4 minutes. Remove the eggs with a slotted spoon and serve on top of the biksemad, sprinkled with chives.

TIP If you like Worcestershire sauce, add a couple of spoonfuls to the mix and serve with organic ketchup.

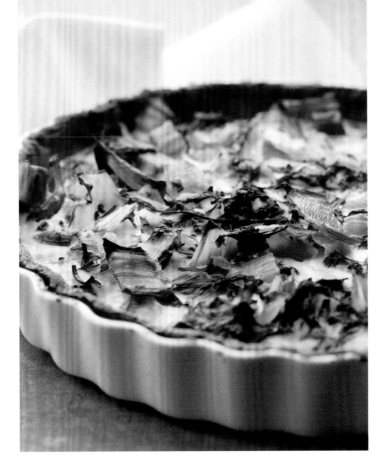

Swiss chard tart

The chard can easily be replaced with broccoli, a very healthy vegetable—and we have grown to think of it as our own here in the North. My great uncle grew broccoli in his garden and he called it asparagus cabbage. SERVES 4

pie dough
½ cup wheat flour
1¾ cups rye flour
1 tsp sea salt flakes
6 tbsp butter
½ cup quark

filling
1 ¾ lbs Swiss chard
canola or olive oil
4 scallions, sliced
4 eggs
⅔ cup quark
scant 1 cup cottage cheese
1 tbsp fresh thyme
1 tsp sea salt flakes
freshly ground pepper

First make the pie dough: Mix the flours and the salt together in a large bowl, then crumble the butter in with your hands. Mix in the quark and bring together as a dough. Knead the dough with your hands. (If you have a food processor, place all of the ingredients into it and blend until it becomes smooth dough.) Let rest in the refrigerator for 30 minutes.

Preheat the oven to 350°F. Roll out the dough and use to line a tart dish, cover with baking parchment, and add some dried beans or rice. Bake blind in the oven for 15 minutes.

While the pie dough is baking, rinse the chard well and cut it into pieces. Heat some oil in a pan and sauté the chard with the scallions for 5 minutes. Drain in a colander.

Beat the eggs in a large bowl, add the quark, cottage cheese, thyme, salt and pepper, then the chard. Remove the beans or rice and the paper from the tart base. Pour the egg mix into the tart base and bake again in the oven for 30 minutes.

Serve warm with a green salad.

TIP This is perfect when served with smoked salmon.

Leek and goat feta tart on rye pie dough

The tart revolution started in the 1970s, and I believe it was partly started in Denmark by the vegetarian restaurant chain Cranks, which opened a café in the center of Copenhagen. I loved their savory tarts with all kinds of vegetables. I still cook a lot of tarts, but I make a dough using quark and rye flour and I also use a low-fat dairy product instead of cream. SERVES 4

pie dough
½ cup wheat flour
1¾ cups rye flour
1 tsp salt flakes
6 tbsp butter
½ cup quark or fromage frais

filling
5 thin leeks, cut into slices
1 tsp salt flakes
4 eggs
⅔ cup quark or fromage frais
5 oz goat feta cheese
1 tbsp chopped fresh thyme
salt and freshly ground pepper

Begin by making the pie dough: Sift the flours and the salt together into a bowl, then crumble the butter in with your hands. Mix in the quark or fromage frais. Knead the resulting dough with your hands. Alternatively, place everything in the food processor and blend it together. If the dough does not come together, add a little water. Let rest in the refrigerator for 30 minutes.

Toward the end of this time, preheat the oven to 350°F. Roll the dough out and use to line a 9½-inch tart dish, then cover with baking parchment and add some dried beans or rice to weigh it down. Bake in the preheated oven for 15 minutes. Remove the paper with the beans or rice and bake again for 5 minutes more.

While the tart case is in the oven, rinse the leeks well (see below). Steam these in a covered sauté pan with a little salted water for about 10 minutes. Drain in a colander.

Beat the eggs in a mixing bowl and add the quark or fromage frais and the feta cheese, then mix in the thyme and the leeks. Pour the mixture into the prebaked tart and place back in the oven. Bake for 30 minutes. Serve warm with a green salad.

TIPS A slice of this tart makes a perfect lunch to take to work. One of the best ways to rinse leeks is first to cut them in slices and then put them in a bowl of cold water and leave for 5 minutes. Lift out of the water so the grit stays at the bottom of the bowl. Sometimes you need to do this twice.

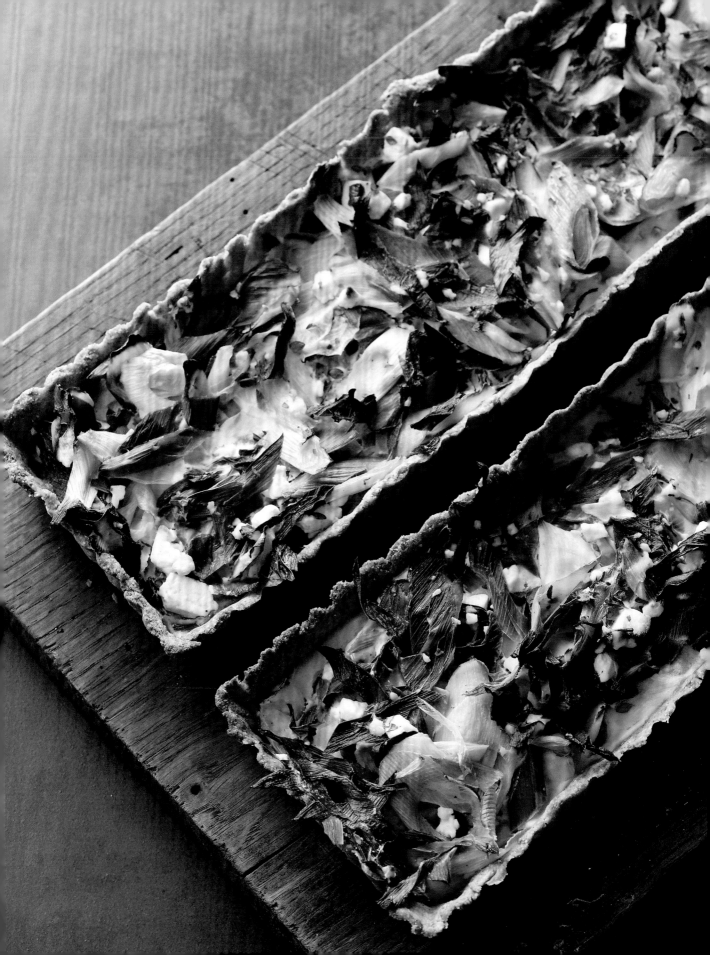

Fish and Shellfish

We must try to eat fish at least twice a week, because fish is such a healthy food. As well as being low in calories and saturated fats, and high in protein, it is rich in a wide range of vitamins and minerals. Oily fish, such as herring, mackerel, salmon, sardines, and tuna, are also good sources of the crucial omega-3 fatty acids, which keep our hearts and our brains healthy and are quite hard to come by in other foods. The Nordic region has, I believe, some of best fish in the world, but of course I would say that and I really think that all countries or areas near the sea have incredible local fish. We should try as much as possible to eat local fish that have not traveled too far and are available to us during their correct (nonbreeding) season. It is also important to try fish that may not be fashionable to eat, but have great potential.

Monkfish cheeks, fennel, and light mash

Monkfish cheeks are very tender and firm pieces of fish that have a wonderful taste, are easy to prepare, and need very little handling—just pan-fry them gently in a little butter. Fennel contains an excellent range of nutrients including vitamin C and folate, and helps the body absorb vital iron. Fennel is also a renowned and useful diuretic. SERVES 4

1 head of fennel
1¼–1½ lbs monkfish cheeks
a little bit of butter
salt and freshly ground pepper
1 tsp fennel seeds

light mash

1¼ lbs unpeeled small potatoes,
  well scrubbed
1 tbsp extra virgin canola oil
2 scallions, chopped
2 sprigs of dill, to garnish

Cook the potatoes in salted boiling water. When just tender, drain them and place them in a bowl. Cover and set aside.

Using a mandoline grater, slice the fennel super thin. Put in cold water.

Prepare the monkfish cheeks: Remove the thin membrane on one side of each cheek and pan-fry the cheeks in butter for 3–4 minutes on each side, until tender. (Cooking time depends on how big they are, so keep an eye on them.) Sprinkle with salt and pepper. Remove the cheeks from the pan when done and keep warm.

Add the fennel seeds and the well-drained fennel to the pan and sauté for 3–4 minutes. Sprinkle with salt and pepper, while the fennel is cooking.

Mash the potatoes roughly with a big balloon whisk, then add the oil, scallions, salt, and pepper. The mash should be very lumpy.

Serve the fish on top of the fennel, and add some fresh dill sprigs on the top of the monkfish cheeks. Serve with the mash.

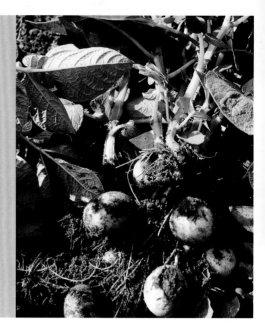

POTATOES have for centuries been the most important basic food for millions of people in our part of the world because of their high energy level. There are a large number of varieties, each country having its favorites. As they are available all year and because we eat so many, they are an important element of nutrition. They are the cheapest source of vitamins B6 and C, potassium, and fiber, and small new potatoes tend to have more nutrients by weight. Especially when eaten with the skin, they provide a great deal of vital dietary fiber. Always store potatoes in a cool, dry place. Potatoes exposed to bright light turn green and become toxic—don't eat them!

Fishcakes with baked potatoes and asparagus

Fishcakes are a big part of Nordic food tradition. They are prepared in many different ways; restaurants even have their "signature" fishcakes, and fish shops sell a wide variety of them. I cook all kinds of different fishcakes, some with salmon, others with cod, haddock, or pollack. They are wonderful as everyday food for dinner, or cold with rye bread for lunch. SERVES 4

1 lb 2 oz skinless, boneless salmon
1 tsp sea salt
2 tbsp oatmeal
2 tbsp flour
whites of 2 eggs
4 tbsp finely grated carrot
4 tbsp coarsely grated squash
1 tbsp minced lemon thyme
1 tbsp canola oil, for pan-frying
1½ tbsp butter, for pan-frying

baked potatoes and asparagus

1 ¼ lbs small potatoes
2 tbsp olive oil
salt and freshly ground pepper
1 bunch of green asparagus
1 organic lemon, cut into wedges

sauce

generous 1 cup yogurt
6 tbsp minced parsley
2 tbsp minced mint leaves

Well ahead, blend the salmon in a food processor. Place it in a bowl, add the teaspoon of sea salt, and stir well, then stir in the remaining ingredients. Place the mixture in the refrigerator to chill for 1 hour.

Preheat the oven to 400°F. Prepare the potatoes for baking: Put them in an ovenproof dish, drizzle with olive oil, sprinkle with salt and pepper, and mix well. Bake in the oven for 30–40 minutes, until tender.

Put the asparagus and lemon pieces in another ovenproof dish and sprinkle with a little salt and pepper. Bake them with the potatoes for their last 8 minutes in the oven.

Using a spoon and your free hand, shape the salmon mixture into balls, then pat gently into flattish rounds. Heat the oil and butter in a skillet and cook the fishcakes over medium heat for 5 minutes on each side.

Meanwhile, make the sauce by mixing the ingredients and season to taste with salt and pepper.

Serve the fishcakes with the potatoes and asparagus, with the sauce served separately.

TIP The salmon can be replaced with either pollack or cod.

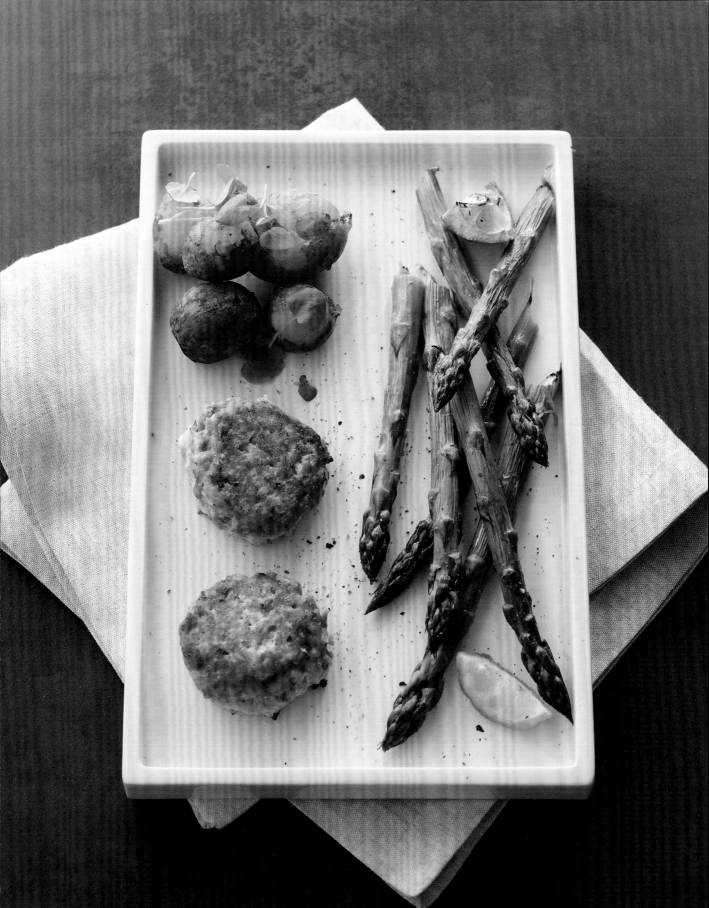

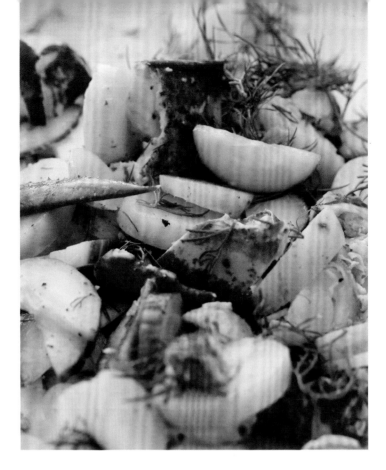

Lobster salad

Although lobsters are caught all year round they are so expensive it makes them a true treat. We also have crayfish and langoustine caught in different regions of the North, and all are part of many different local food traditions. Like fish, most shellfish are a low-calorie and low-saturated fat source of protein. They are also rich in a wide array of vitamins and minerals, including the antioxidants vitamin E and selenium, which are both otherwise difficult to find in most average diets. SERVES 4

2 live lobsters, each about 1 lb 2 oz

brine
1 tbsp coarse sea salt
1 tbsp whole peppercorns
3 dill stalks

salad
14 oz boiled new potatoes
⅓ cucumber, halved and sliced
juice from ½ to 1 unwaxed lemon
1 tbsp extra virgin olive oil
2 sprigs of dill, chopped
salt and freshly ground pepper

First make the brine: Add 5¼ quarts of water to a large pot together with the salt, peppercorns, and dill. Bring to a boil. When the brine is boiling, place the lobster in the brine, cover with a lid, and let it boil for 7 minutes. Remove the lobster from the pan and let cool.

When cool, crack open and get the lobster meat. First break off the head, then break off the claws. Take the tail, cut it in half lengthwise, then crack open the claws and remove all the lobster meat, place on a plate, and set aside.

To make the salad, cut the potatoes into thin slices. In a big salad bowl, mix the potatoes, cucumber, lemon juice, olive oil, dill, and lots of pepper. Then cut the lobster meat into smaller pieces and gently mix into the salad. Season with salt.

Serve the salad right away.

TIP Always buy live lobster, as once dead they decompose very rapidly. The most humane way to deal with them is to put them in the freezer for a few hours before cooking as they then go into a deep sleep.

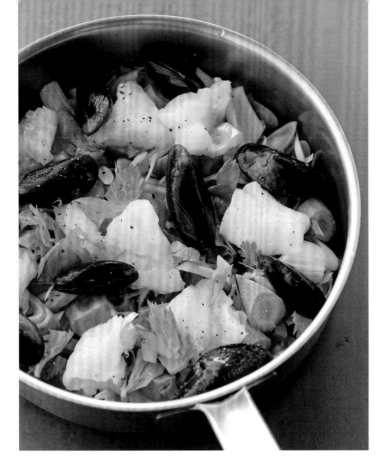

Mussel and cod stew with vegetables and white wine

This fish stew is tasty and easy to make. Once you've assembled everything, it takes just 10 minutes to cook it and for it to be ready to eat. Mussels are one of the few types of shellfish that are rich in omega-3s, as well as being packed with vitamins and minerals. SERVES 4

1 lb 2 oz mussels
2 celery stalks, cut into slices
2 carrots, cut into chunks
2 leeks, well rinsed and cut across
  into slices
salt and freshly ground pepper
generous ¾ cup white wine
1 lb 2 oz skinless cod fillets, broken
  into small pieces
spelt bread, to serve

Scrub the mussels thoroughly and tug out any beards that may be hanging from the shells. Discard any broken or open mussels or those that refuse to close when the shell is tapped. Rinse the mussels in cold water a couple of times.

In a large sauté pan, place the celery, carrots, and leeks, then sprinkle with salt and pepper. Place the mussels in between and on top of the vegetables. Pour the white wine over the fish and vegetables. Cover with a lid and bring to a boil, then turn down the heat and let it simmer for 5 minutes.

Remove the lid and place the cod in between the mussels, sprinkle with salt and pepper, and let it simmer again for 5 minutes.

Serve from the sauté pan with spelt bread.

TIP If you don't like mussels, then make the stew without and just add a bit more cod.

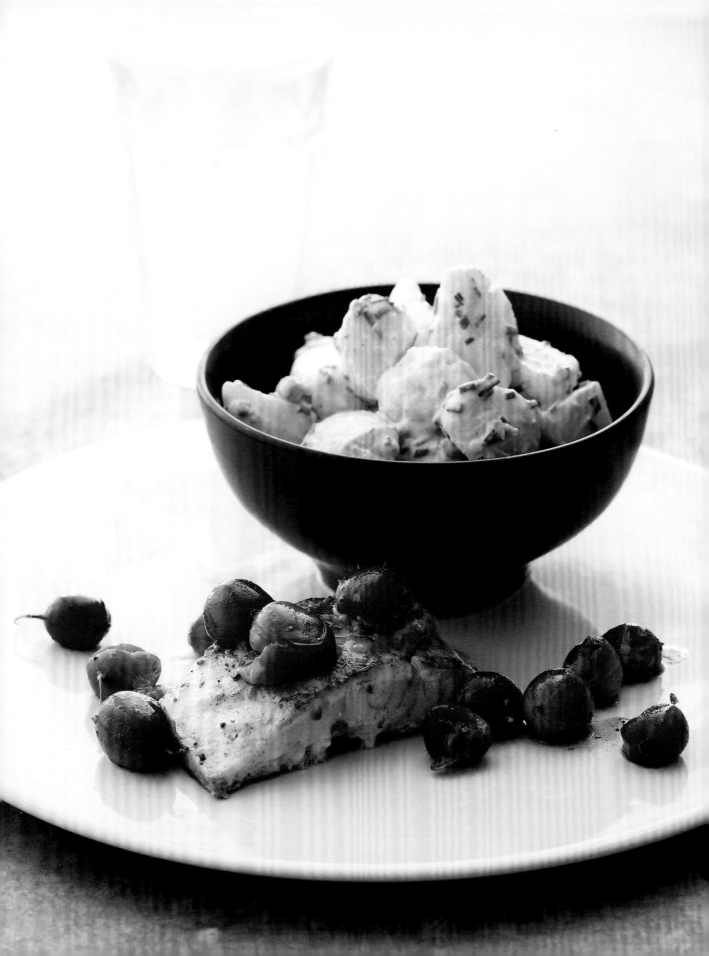

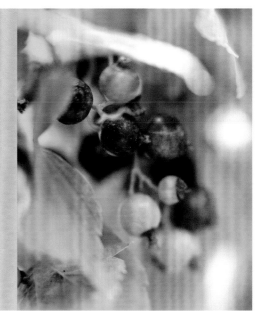

GOOSEBERRIES grow wild and are cultivated widely across Northern Europe. Although the green ones with the fuzzy skins are the most familiar, there are many varieties in different colors—white, yellow, and red—and often with smooth skins. Closely related to the black currant and red currant, they also vary in their degree of sweetness; some are sweet enough to eat raw, but most need stewing with sugar. They have long been held to be good for digestion and the liver, as well as helping alleviate arthritis. They are rich in vitamin C and fiber, and are a good source of vitamin A, potassium, and manganese. Phytochemicals in them are thought to help protect against heart disease and to be antidepressants.

Pan-fried mullet with gooseberries and potato salad

Mullet is a perfect summer fish that is easy to broil because its flesh is nice and firm. It goes well with the tasty but sour gooseberries. SERVES 4

2 gray mullet fillets,
  each about 14 oz
1 cup red gooseberries
1½ tbsp butter

potato salad
14 oz new potatoes
2 tbsp low-fat yogurt
2 tbsp Dijon mustard
4 tbsp chopped dill
2 tbsp capers
salt and freshly ground pepper
1 cup shelled peas

Start by making the potato salad: Cook the new potatoes in salted boiling water, drain, and then let them cool down.

In a mixing bowl, mix the yogurt, mustard, dill, and capers well and season to taste with salt and pepper. Cut the cooled potatoes into chunks, add to the dressing together with the peas, and mix in gently.

Cut the mullet fillets into pieces. Rinse the gooseberries and drain.

Melt the butter in a skillet and pan-fry the mullet fillets skin side down for 2 minutes, then turn the fillets over and add the gooseberries. Let pan-fry for 5–7 minutes. Sprinkle with salt and pepper.

Serve right away with the potato salad.

TIPS Late in the season you can use lingonberries in place of the gooseberries, but then add ¼ cup of sugar as well.

If you want to broil mullet, brush the fillets with oil on both sides and broil at medium heat for a couple of minutes, then sprinkle with salt and pepper.

Savoy fish rolls with spelt salad

This makes a very green-colored meal that is also very light. SERVES 4

8 big leaves of a savoy cabbage
8 plaice fillets, each about 5 oz
salt and freshly ground pepper
generous ¾ cup white wine

filling

1 tsp canola oil
½ leek, chopped
½ squash, diced
10 sprigs of lemon thyme, chopped
2 tbsp grainy mustard, plus more
   to serve

spelt salad

5 oz spelt kernels
11 oz green beans
3½ oz arugula
2 tbsp white wine vinegar
1 tbsp olive oil
salt and freshly ground
   pepper

Cook the cabbage leaves in salted boiling water for 5 minutes, remove, and drain them well.

Make the filling: Heat the oil in a sauté pan, then add the leek, squash, and lemon thyme. Cook for 5 minutes. Turn off the heat, add the mustard, and mix well. Set aside.

Make the spelt salad: Cook the spelt kernels in salted boiling water for 30 minutes. Drain thoroughly and put in a large bowl. Let it cool down.

Preheat the oven to 350°F. Place the cooled cabbage leaves on a counter and place a fish fillet on each of them. Sprinkle with salt and pepper, then place 1 tablespoon of the filling on them and roll them up. Put them in an ovenproof tray and pour the wine over them. Cover with foil and bake in the preheated oven for 15 minutes.

When the spelt has cooled, add the other ingredients all at the same time, mix well, and season to taste with salt and pepper.

Serve the fish rolls with the salad and some grainy mustard on the side.

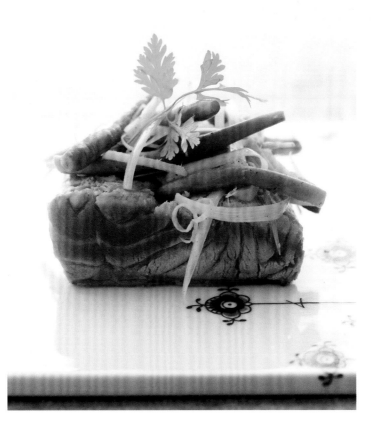

Salmon with carrots, ginger, leeks, green beans, and chervil

Salmon is a very northern hemisphere fish and we eat a lot of it in many different ways: raw, smoked, cold, fried, baked, marinated, or as gravlax. Here I cook the fish in a dry pan, so it cooks in its own oils for a good true flavor. SERVES 4

4 pieces of salmon fillet, about
  1½–1¾ lbs
7 oz baby carrots
1 leek, cut into fine julienne strips
7oz green beans, trimmed of ends
3½ oz fresh ginger, minced
1 bunch of chervil
salt and freshly ground pepper

to serve
green salad
baguette (optional)

Pan-fry the salmon in a hot dry pan for 2–3 minutes on each side. Remove the salmon from the pan, add the vegetables, ginger, and chervil, and let them cook for 5 minutes. Season to taste with salt and pepper.

Place the salmon fillets on a serving platter and spread the cooked vegetables over them. Serve with a green salad and maybe a baguette.

Pointed cabbage forms a bright green narrow, oblong head and is an early vegetable in season from May to August. It has a short development time and is easy to grow but you have to harvest it at the right time as it has a tendency to bolt. It has the same strongly beneficial nutritional qualities as other types of green cabbage.

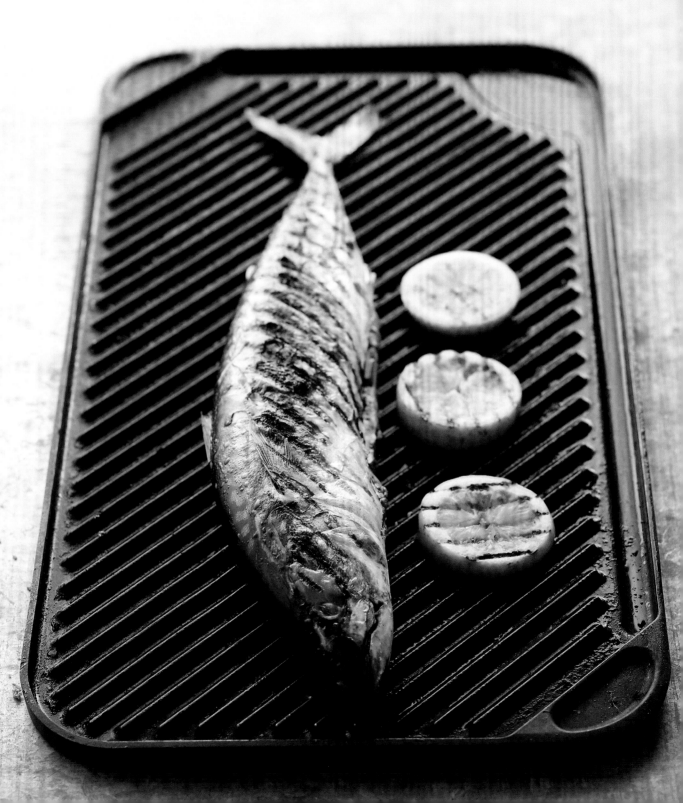

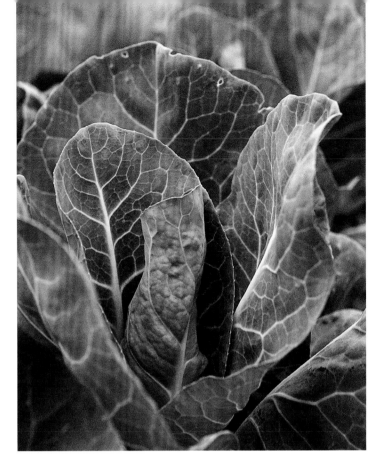

Pan-fried mackerel with baked rhubarb and pointed cabbage

A very oily fish (hence a great provider of the beneficial omega-3 fats), mackerel is very beautiful, with its characteristic black and dark green coloring. It can be caught all year around, but most commonly during spring and summer. In August they are perfect for smoking as their fat content is then at its highest. I serve rhubarb as a savory that goes very well with it. SERVES 4

4 rhubarb stalks
¼ cup sugar (optional)
light vegetable oil, for brushing
2 large whole mackerel,
    each about 1½ lbs
1 unwaxed lemon, sliced
1 pointed cabbage
1½ tbsp butter
salt and freshly ground pepper

to serve
4 slices of spelt or rye bread

Preheat the oven to 350°F and prepare a hot broiler, griddle, or stovetop grill pan.

Cut the rhubarb into pieces about 2 inches thick. Place in an ovenproof dish brushed with a little oil. Bake in the preheated oven for 15 minutes.

While the rhubarb is baking, brush the mackerel with a little oil and broil or griddle for 5–8 minutes on each side and the lemon slices for a couple of minutes on each side.

Cut the cabbage lengthwise into 6 pieces and rinse in cold water. Drain them well.

Heat the butter in a skillet and pan-fry the cabbage on all sides until golden brown and nicely caramelized. Sprinkle with salt and pepper.

Serve the mackerel with the lemon slices, baked rhubarb, pointed cabbage, and some spelt or rye bread.

TIP If you want your rhubarb a little sweeter add the sugar.

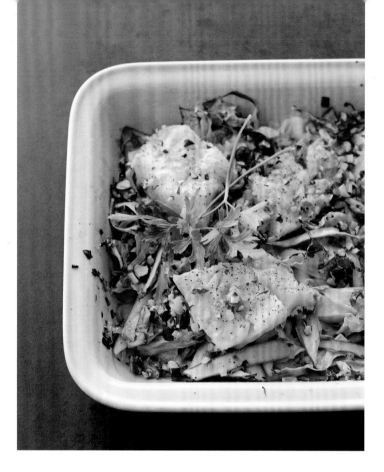

Baked haddock with a lemon gremolata

Like many nuts, almonds are considered a "superfood" as they are so full of good essential nutrients. Use the whole shelled nuts and not the blanched ones, as their skins are highly nutritious. SERVES 4

½ pointed cabbage, shredded
1 bunch of asparagus, cut into slices
   lengthwise
1 head of fennel in thin slices
1¾ lbs skinless boneless haddock fillets
juice from 1 lemon
salt and freshly ground pepper

gremolata
1 tsp canola oil
1 shallot, minced
1 tsp grated zest from an
   unwaxed lemon
⅓ cup almonds, chopped

yogurt sauce
⅔ cup yogurt
juice from ½ lemon
2 tbsp minced parsley

Preheat the oven to 350°F.

Start by making the gremolata: Heat the oil in a skillet and add the shallot, lemon zest, and almonds. Let these cook gently for 2 minutes. Turn out on a dish and set aside.

Put the pointed cabbage, asparagus, and fennel in an ovenproof dish and mix well. Now place the haddock fillets on top. Pour over the lemon juice and sprinkle with salt and pepper. Spread the gremolata over the pieces of fish and bake in the preheated oven for 10 minutes.

Mix the ingredients for the yogurt sauce, seasoning to taste with salt and pepper.

Serve the haddock straight from the dish with the cold yogurt sauce.

Cod with cauliflower in mustard dressing and spelt spinach stew

Do ask your fish supplier or supermarket to ensure that the cod you buy is from a sustainable source. SERVES 6

7 oz spelt kernels
1 lb 2 oz spinach
1 whole cod, about 2¾ lbs
1 onion, cut in half
3 bay leaves
1 tbsp whole peppercorns
1 tbsp sea salt
1 cauliflower, separated into florets
1 tbsp canola oil
1 garlic clove, chopped
salt and freshly ground pepper

mustard dressing
3 tbsp grainy mustard
1 tbsp Dijon mustard
6 tbsp chopped parsley

Boil the spelt in a generous amount of water for 10 minutes, drain, and leave in the strainer. Rinse the spinach well in cold water, remove any tough stems, and drain well.

Cut the cod into large pieces, place in a pan, and add the onion, bay leaves, peppercorns, and salt with just enough water to cover the cod. Bring to a boil. Once boiling, turn off the heat and leave for 10 minutes with the lid on.

Sauté the cauliflower in a dry pan for a couple of minutes; if it starts to stick to the pan add a little water. Season with salt and pepper.

Make the mustard cream by mixing the ingredients, season to taste, and then mix it into the warm cauliflower.

Slowly heat the oil and garlic in another sauté pan and then add the spinach and cook until wilted. Add the cooked spelt and mix well. Season to taste with salt and pepper.

Take the cod out of the water and place on a serving dish. Serve with the spelt and the cauliflower in mustard dressing.

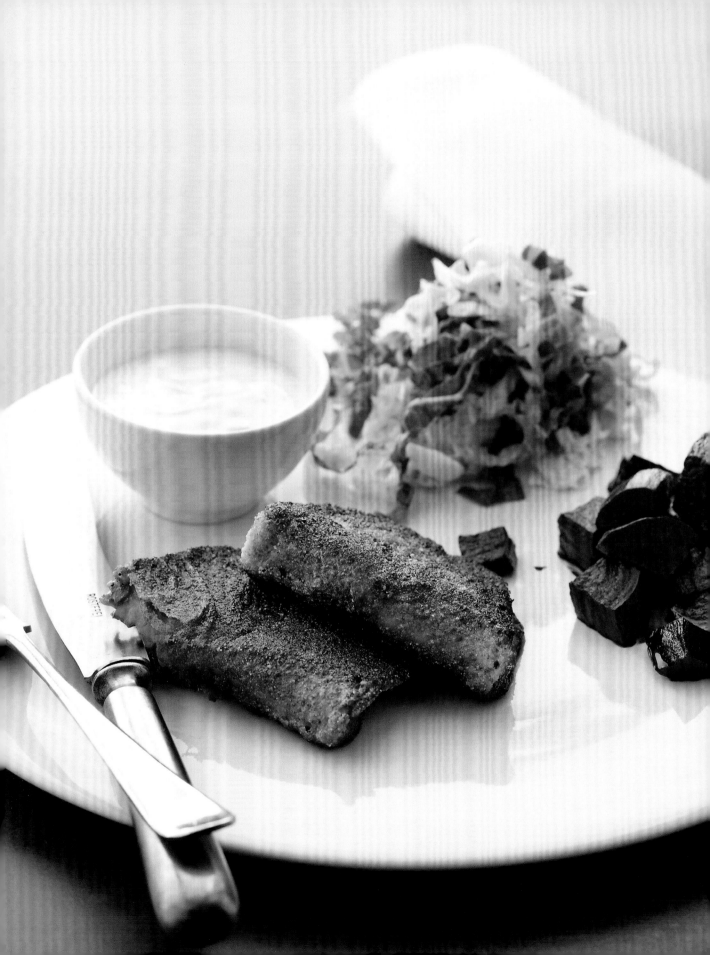

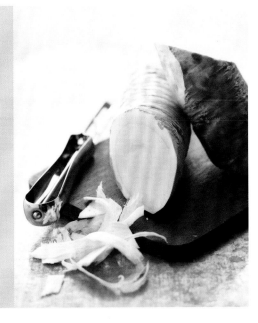

HORSERADISH comes from southeastern Europe and western Asia, but grows well in the Northern European climate. Actually a member of the cabbage family, it is the tap root that we eat. It contains vitamin C, folate, potassium, calcium, iron, magnesium, and phosphorus, as well as mustard oil, which has antibacterial properties. The root is also a good source of isothiocyanates, phytochemicals that have been shown to help against various cancers. The plant grows wild in many places in the countryside. It is perennial and can be harvested as long as the leaves are seen.

Pan-fried herring with beet and horseradish sauce

I love herring as they can be cooked in many different ways. This is a healthy everyday recipe, which is also inexpensive because fresh herrings are not a luxury fish. SERVES 4

8 herring fillets, each about 5 oz
1 cup rye flour
1–2 tbsp canola oil
4 slices of rye bread, to serve

beet
14 oz beets
5 tbsp blueberry cordial
salt and freshly ground pepper

horseradish dressing
generous ¾ cup yogurt
1 tsp honey
2 tsp lime juice
2 oz horseradish, finely grated
2 tbsp capers

green salad
7 oz green salad leaves
juice from ½ lemon

First prepare the beets: peel them and cut them into cubes about ¾ x ¾ inches. Place them in a pan with the blueberry cordial, 5 tablespoons of water, very little salt, and some pepper. Bring to a boil, then cover with a lid and let simmer for 10 minutes. Remove the lid, increase the heat, and, if necessary, fully reduce the juice to a glaze while stirring.

Cut off the little dorsal fin from each herring fillet and rinse. Mix the rye flour, salt, and plenty of pepper. Press the fillets skin-side down in the flour, so they are completely covered, and then fold them over.

Pan-fry in the oil for 4–5 minutes on each side or until golden brown.

Mix all the ingredients for the horseradish sauce, seasoning to taste with salt, pepper, and maybe more lime juice.

Serve the herring with the beet, horseradish dressing, and green salad dressed with lemon juice.

TIP If you can't get fresh herring, use either mackerel or mullet instead.

Game and Poultry

Game has been part of our food culture for centuries, and probably for thousands of years before we actually farmed animals. Primitive man would hunt wild animals and cook them over an open fire. Today we eat far more farmed animals, and much more than our bodies really need. For reasons both of our health and the domino effect it has on climate change, we need to start cutting down on the amount of meat we eat. However, meat is still a tasty treat, an important source of protein, and an essential part of a lot of classic and wonderful recipes. Therefore, when we plan our diet we should reduce overall meat consumption and also start including game in our food, as being mostly wild and more seasonal, there is less waste included in its production. Moreover, animals that live and eat in their natural habitat have leaner meat with a wider range of nutrients and few of the growth-promoting and medicinal additives found in reared meat.

Summer deer with rhubarb-ginger chutney

In early summer we get the tender fillets from the young summer bucks, which are culled at this time of year. The season in Denmark is from June 16 to July 16. I serve this with summer vegetables and chutney instead of a sauce. SERVES 6

1¼ lbs new potatoes
salt and freshly ground pepper
4 leeks, cut into 2-inch lengths and
    rinsed well
1 summer buck venison fillet (use lamb
    fillet or chicken breast if unavailable)
2 tbsp butter
chopped chervil, to serve

rhubarb-ginger chutney
11 oz rhubarb, cut into small pieces
3½ oz fresh ginger, grated
1 tbsp whole peppercorns
about ½ cup sugar
1 tbsp white wine vinegar

Place all the ingredients for the chutney in a pan and simmer for 20 minutes. Season and add more sugar to taste, if necessary. Let it cool down. Store in sterilized jars and serve with game and poultry dishes.

Cook the potatoes in salted boiling water until just tender and steam the leeks in salted water for 4 minutes. Drain both and keep warm.

Melt the butter in a skillet, pan-fry the fillet in the butter for about 5 minutes each side until nicely colored, then sprinkle with salt and pepper.

Cut the meat into slices, scatter the chervil on top, and serve with the vegetables and chutney.

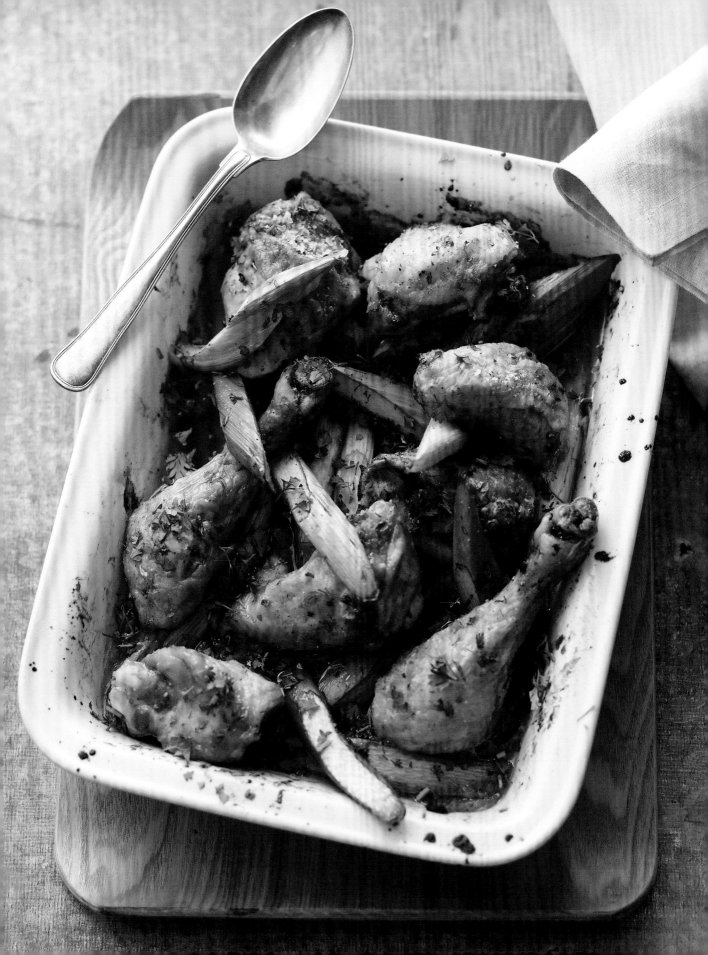

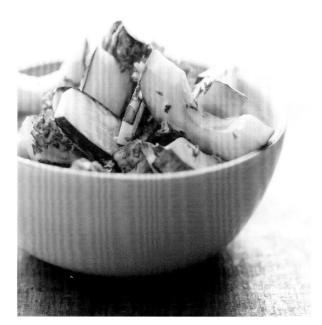

Chicken with baked rhubarb and cucumber-radish salad

Rhubarb and chicken make a perfect match and a very tasty spring dish when the rhubarb is in season. Rhubarb is also fantastic as a savory vegetable. SERVES 4

1 organic or free-range chicken,
  cut into 8 pieces
salt and freshly ground pepper
11 oz rhubarb
¼ cup raw organic sugar

cucumber-radish salad
1 cucumber, seeded and sliced
1 bunch of radishes, sliced

dressing
generous ⅓ cup goat-milk yogurt
1 garlic clove, minced
2 tbsp chopped mint

Preheat the oven to 400°F. Put the chicken pieces in an ovenproof dish, sprinkle with salt and pepper, and roast in the preheated oven for 30 minutes.

Cut the rhubarb into pieces and mix it with the sugar in a bowl.

Take the chicken out of the oven, place the rhubarb under the chicken, put it back in the oven, and roast for 15 minutes more.

Make the salad: Mix the cucumber and radish slices in a bowl. Blend together the dressing ingredients and mix this into the salad. Season with salt and pepper.

Serve the chicken and rhubarb with the salad and boiled potatoes.

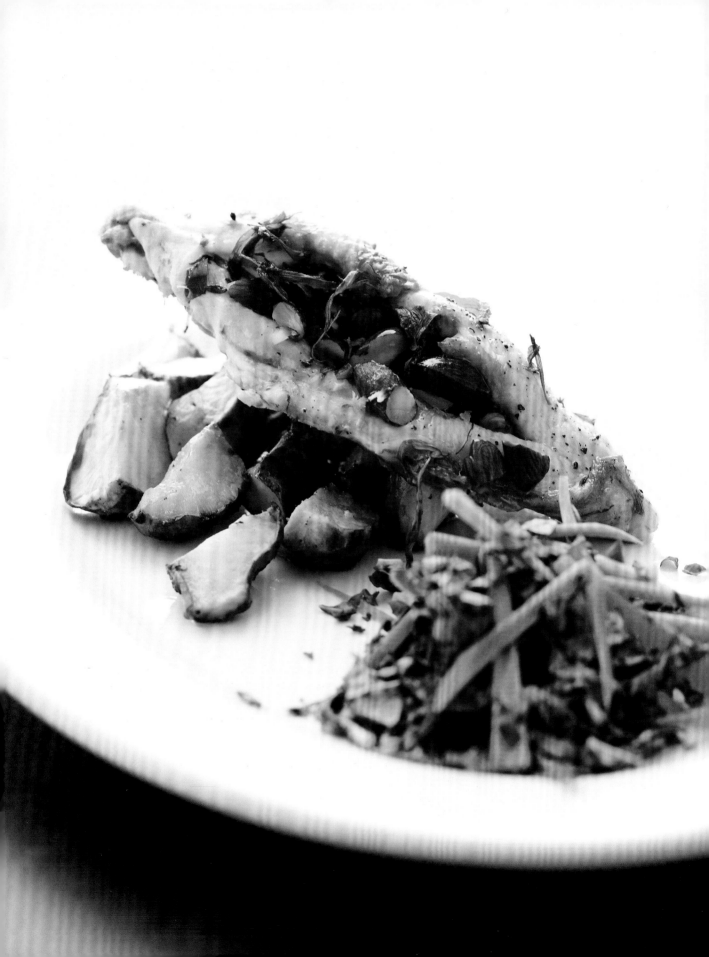

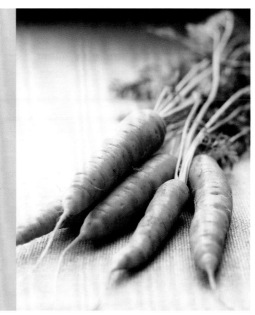

CARROTS are packed with antioxidants, as they are the richest food source of beta-carotene, which the body converts to vitamin A. This is even more readily available when the carrot is cooked. They are also a good source of fiber, various B vitamins, vitamins C and K, potassium, and manganese. Although nowadays the bright orange carrot is the most familiar, they can be white, purple, or yellow. There are early and late varieties, so the season is from June for forced carrots, July to September for early outdoor-grown carrots, October and November for the main crop, and December onward for the late main crops. As they are easy to store, carrots are available all year round.

Tarragon chicken with Jerusalem artichokes and kale and carrot salad

Tarragon is one of my favorite herbs. I use it with chicken, in salads and fishcakes, and in dressings. I grow tarragon in my front yard in a large pot, which I move to my kitchen window in winter. SERVES 4

4 organic or free-range chicken
  breasts on the bone
⅓ cup almonds, chopped
8 tbsp chopped fresh tarragon
½ tsp salt
1¼ lbs Jerusalem artichokes
3 garlic cloves, halved
2 tbsp olive oil
salt and freshly ground pepper

kale salad
11 oz kale
3 carrots

dressing
1 tbsp Dijon mustard
2 tbsp apple cider vinegar
1 tbsp walnut oil

Preheat the oven to 400°F. Cut a pocket in the side of each chicken breast for the filling.

In a bowl, mix the almonds, tarragon, and salt. Stuff this filling into the pockets you've made in the chicken.

Cut the Jerusalem artichokes into chunks and place in a big ovenproof dish with the garlic. Mix in the olive oil, salt, and pepper. Place the chicken breasts on top of the Jerusalem artichokes and bake in the preheated oven for 25 minutes.

To prepare the kale salad, remove the tough stems from the leaves and rinse the leaves in cold water. Drain in a colander and then mince. Cut the carrots into julienne strips and mix with the kale.

Whisk the dressing ingredients together and mix into the salad just before serving.

Serve the chicken breasts with the Jerusalem artichokes and the kale salad.

TIP The almonds can be replaced with hazelnuts.

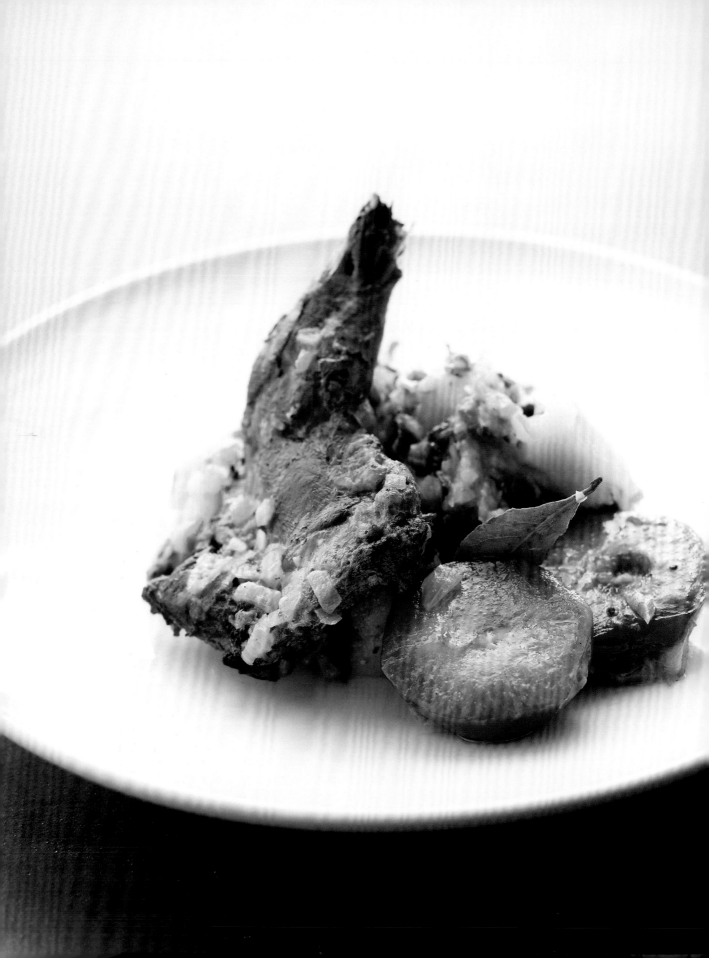

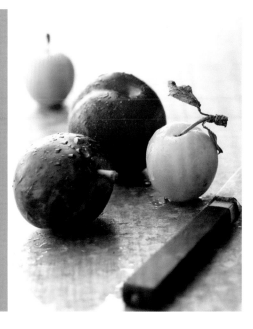

PLUMS, the second-most cultivated fruit in the world, are a good source of fiber, potassium, and vitamins A and C. The dark-skinned varieties contain useful amounts of beta-carotene, which is an important antioxidant phytochemical that is also thought to help fight some cancers. Dried plums—prunes—are known for their laxative effect, and regular intake has been shown to lower (bad) LDL cholesterol in the blood and may even help against colon cancer. Plums mature in August and September, depending on the variety.

Braised pheasant, plums, and kale mash

Pheasants are tricky, as they can be very dull if overcooked. The meat is different every time I cook it, so my best advice is to look after it and take nothing for granted. Cooking is like everything else in life: The more you do it, the better you become at it. Fresh pheasant is the best and, when you get it right, it is food made in heaven, with lots of flavor, texture, and tenderness. If you don't feel up to the challenge, this dish works equally well with chicken and rabbit pieces. SERVES 4

1 tbsp olive oil
2 pheasants, each cut into 4 pieces
2 garlic cloves, chopped
1 onion, chopped
3 bay leaves
1 big bunch of parsley, chopped
1¼ cups white wine
1 lb 2 oz plums, halved and pitted

mash
1¼ lbs potatoes, cut into chunks
3½ oz kale, chopped
1 tbsp canola oil
salt and freshly ground pepper

Heat the oil in a pan and brown the pheasant all over. Add the garlic, onion, bay, and parsley. Cook for 3 minutes. Add the wine, season, and simmer for 15 minutes. Add the plums and simmer for 15 minutes more.

While the pheasant is cooking, boil the potatoes in salted boiling water for 20 minutes or until tender. For the last 5 minutes of cooking, add the chopped kale, then drain but save some of the vegetable water.

Place the potatoes and kale in a mixing bowl and use a balloon whisk to mash them. Add the oil and mix it in, then add a little of the reserved cooking water to the mash for a nice smooth finish. Season to taste.

Serve the pheasant with the cooked plums and the kale mash.

TIP Mash is perfect for winter as boiled winter potatoes are mealy and a bit lacking in flavor, while mash can be mixed with any vegetable you like. You can even use leftover boiled vegetables from the day before, and you don't have to add butter or whole milk, just a little (nicely flavored) oil, and use the vegetable water or skim milk.

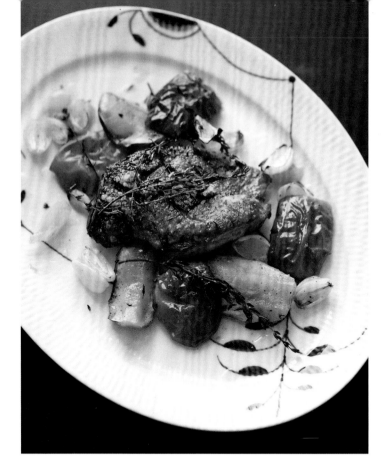

Goose breast with apples and celeriac salad

Goose is traditional at Christmas in a lot of households. In my house we eat duck, which means that I do not eat a whole goose very often, but only as an alternative, and then I will just cook a goose breast. SERVES 4

2 goose breasts
2 onions, quartered
4 Pippin apples, cored
  and cut into chunks
10 sprigs of thyme
salt and freshly ground pepper

celeriac salad

14 oz celeriac
4 tbsp yogurt
2 tbsp Dijon mustard
4 tbsp chopped lovage

Preheat the oven to 400°F. Score the skin on top of the breast in a lattice pattern. Place the onions, apples, and thyme in an ovenproof dish, put the goose breasts on top, and sprinkle with salt and pepper. Place in the preheated oven and cook for 18 minutes.

To make the celeriac salad: Peel the celeriac and, using a mandolin grater, cut it into thin julienne strips. Mix the remaining ingredients and then stir in the celeriac. Season to taste with salt and pepper.

Carve the goose breasts into slices and serve with apples and onion, and the salad.

TIP Instead of goose breast you can use duck breast and in place of celeriac you could also use carrots or white cabbage.

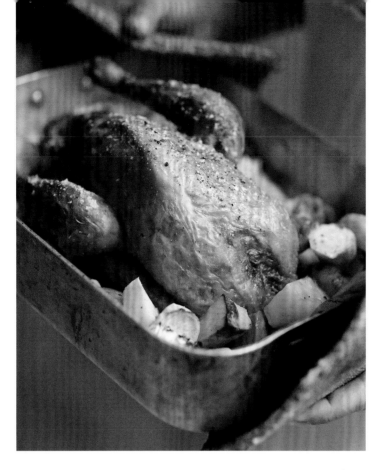

Roast guinea fowl with lemon verbena

I really enjoy guinea fowl and eat them often. I really like the slightly gamey taste of the meat, and it is a perfect substitute for chicken. I also eat the breast with salad or in a quick stir-fry. SERVES 4–6

2 guinea fowl
1 bunch of parsley
2 garlic cloves
2–3 sprigs of lemon verbena
salt and freshly ground pepper
a fall salad (page 55),
  to serve

vegetables

2 carrots
7 oz parsley root or celeriac
  (see page 103)
7 oz Jerusalem artichokes

Preheat the oven to 400°F. Stuff the birds with the parsley, garlic, and lemon verbena, then sprinkle with salt and pepper.

Peel all the vegetables and cut them into chunks. Place in an ovenproof dish, sprinkle with salt and pepper, and place the birds on top. Roast in the preheated oven for 1 hour.

Take out of the oven, cut each bird into 6 pieces, and serve with the root vegetables and a fall salad.

TIPS If you serve this to 4 people, there should be some leftovers for a sandwich the next day. Instead of guinea fowl you can use a large organic chicken, but cook it for about 20 minutes longer.

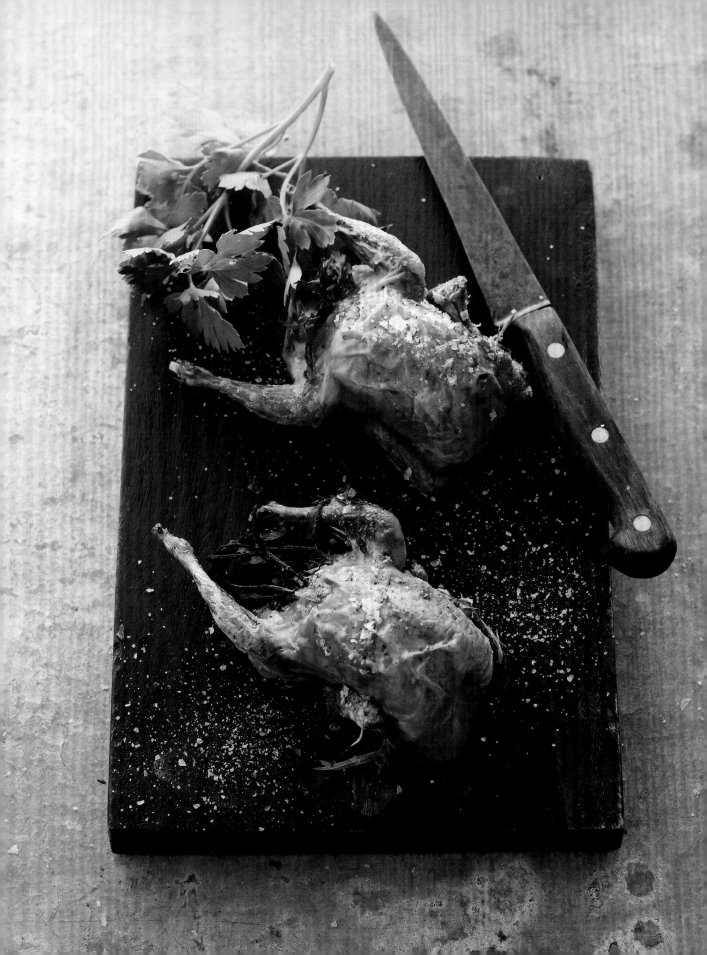

PARSLEY ROOT, or turnip-rooted parsley, is closely related to parsley but has a root that resembles a parsnip or white carrot. These are rich in antioxidant vitamin C and minerals. The soil must be well cultivated before sowing, so it is easy to grow. Harvest from September until the frost comes, then store in a dry, cold place.

Quail with salsify and savoy cabbage

These tasty little birds are perfect for supper on a Saturday night. One is enough for me, but some might think it is too little meat. However, that is what we need to get used to—less meat, more vegetables. SERVES 4

4 quails
1 big bunch of Italian parsley
4 garlic cloves, halved
salt and freshly ground pepper
12 salsify
milk, to cover
1 savoy cabbage
1 tbsp olive oil

mash

7 oz parsley root or parsnips,
   cut into chunks
7 oz carrots, cut into chunks
11 oz large potatoes, peeled and
   cut into chunks
2 tbsp extra virgin olive oil
salt and freshly ground pepper

Preheat the oven to 400°F. Stuff the birds with the parsley and garlic, sprinkle with salt and pepper, and place in an ovenproof dish. Bake in the preheated oven for 25 minutes.

Start making the mash: Cook the parsley root or parsnips, carrots, and potatoes in salted boiling water for 20 minutes, or until tender.

Drain, reserving a little of the cooking water, and place these vegetables in a mixing bowl. Use a balloon whisk to mash the vegetables. Add the olive oil and a little bit of the vegetable water, season to taste with salt and pepper, and keep warm.

Peel the salsify and cut into small pieces. Place them in milk until you have to use them. Cut the cabbage into thin slices.

Add the oil to a pan, then sauté the salsify and cabbage until tender, about 6–7 minutes. Season to taste with salt and pepper.

Serve the quail with this and the mash right away.

TIPS Instead of savoy cabbage, you can use either kale or broccoli. Instead of quail you can use Cornish hens.

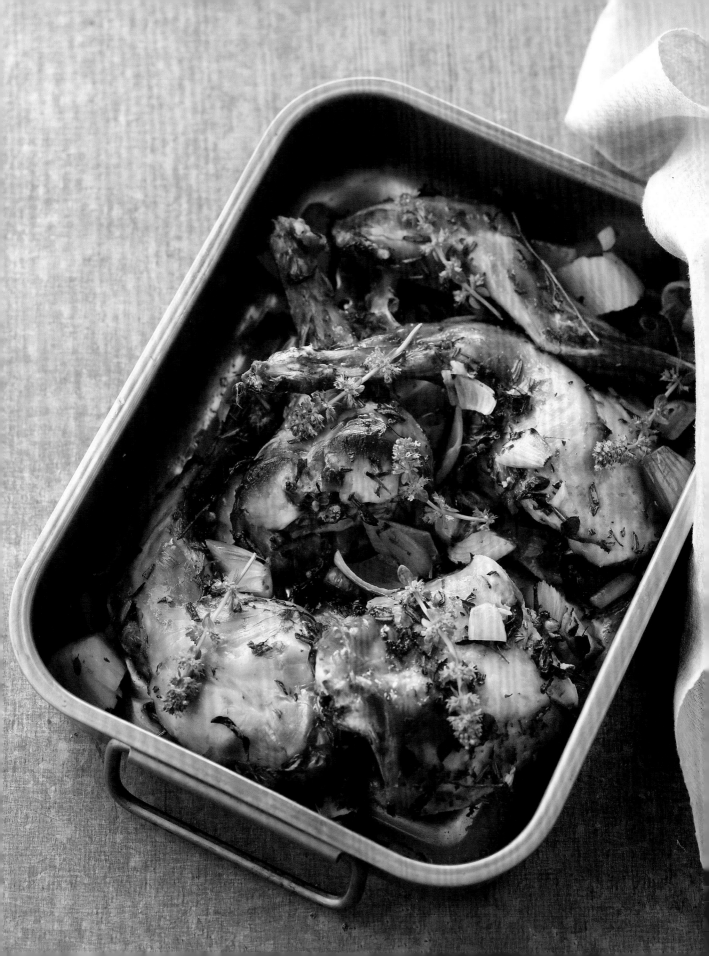

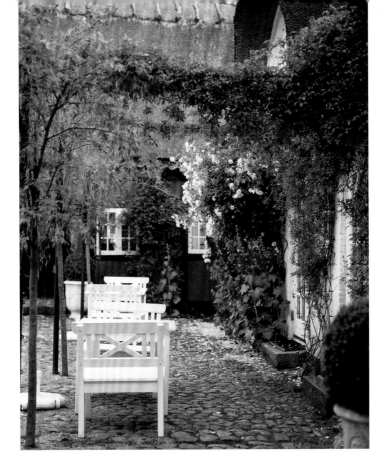

Rabbit stew with rosemary and lemon

Rabbit is widely available again and very tasty, especially when wild. We make a choice to eat meat, but we should eat less, as we don't need to eat meat every day, and it will help protect the planet from climate change. Eating wild food—that is already available naturally—makes more sense to me. Furthermore, it tastes fantastic. SERVES 6

1 dressed rabbit

herb paste
4 garlic cloves, chopped
grated zest of 1 unwaxed lemon
2 tbsp each chopped thyme,
   marjoram, and rosemary
salt and freshly ground pepper
a little olive oil

vegetable stew
1 tbsp olive oil
3 shallots, chopped
2 celery stalks, cut into slices
1 squash, cut into cubes

green salad and spelt bread (page 138),
   to serve

Cut the rabbit into 8 pieces, then make the herb paste by mixing all the ingredients except the olive oil. Rub the rabbit in the mixture and leave in the refrigerator for 2 hours.

Preheat the oven to 350°F. Drizzle the rabbit with a little olive oil. Place in an ovenproof dish and roast in the preheated oven for 30 minutes.

Make the vegetable stew: Heat the olive oil in a pan, add the shallots, celery, squash, and salt and pepper. Cook for 5 minutes.

Place the rabbit on a serving dish, spread the vegetables over the rabbit, and serve with a green salad and spelt bread.

TIP Rabbit meat is white and tender, and, like chicken, can overcook easily. It is actually a lot like chicken, so if you can't get rabbit make the same recipes with chicken.

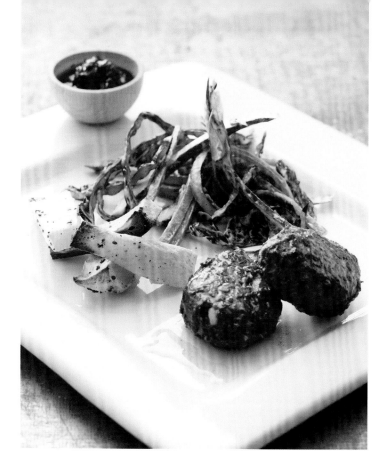

Venison meatballs with baked root veg

Venison is well suited to meatballs. If you can't get venison, you can make the meatballs with lamb. SERVES 4–6

1¼ lbs ground venison
2 eggs
1⅓ cups oats
½ cup rye flour
10 juniper berries, crushed
3 carrots
1 onion, minced
salt and freshly ground pepper
14 oz parsley root (page 103)
14 oz parsnips
2 tbsp virgin olive oil
1 tsp anise, lightly crushed
1 tbsp canola oil, for pan-frying
14 oz red cabbage
½ cup walnuts
2 tbsp raspberry vinegar
generous ¾ cup yogurt (1% fat)
lingonberry compote (page 110)

Make the meatballs: In a bowl, mix together the venison, eggs, oats, flour, juniper, one of the carrots, shredded, and the onion. Season to taste and let the mixture rest in the refrigerator for 30 minutes.

To prepare the baked root vegetables, peel the parsley root and parsnips, and cut them lengthwise, then place them in an ovenproof dish, mix in the olive oil, anise, and salt and pepper to taste.

Preheat the oven to 350°F. Take the chilled meat mixture out of the refrigerator and use a spoon and your free hand to shape the meat mixture into about 24 small round balls.

Pan-fry these in a very little oil in a skillet until they are golden brown on all sides. Place in an ovenproof dish and finish in the preheated oven for 20 minutes, together with the prepared root vegetables.

While these are in the oven, prepare the salad: Cut the red cabbage into very thin slices and the remaining carrots into julienne strips, then mix the cabbage, carrots, and walnuts. In another bowl, mix the vinegar and yogurt, then add to the salad and mix well. Season to taste with salt and pepper.

Serve the meatballs with the baked root vegetables, salad, and lingonberry compote.

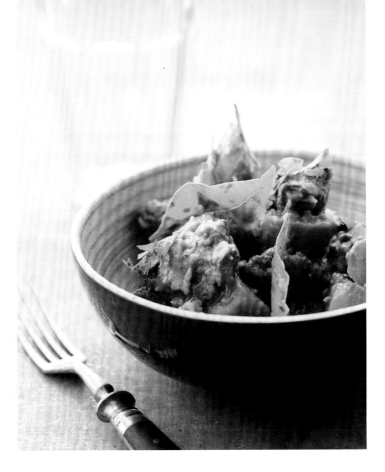

Venison and mushroom stew

Venison stew is very tasty, but you need to be careful not to overcook it, as the lean deer meat can get very dry and lose its full flavor. Use the shoulder or the rump from deer, roe deer, or moose. SERVES 4

1½ tbsp butter
1¼ lbs venison (see above),
   cut into ¾-inch squares
2 tbsp all-purpose flour
12 juniper berries, crushed
2 garlic cloves, chopped
3 bay leaves
5 sprigs of thyme
7 oz baby onions, peeled
1¼ cups red wine
11 oz mushrooms, chopped
3 carrots, cut into cubes
14 oz parsley root (page 103),
   peeled and cut into cubes
salt and freshly ground pepper

to serve
1¼ lbs potatoes, boiled
2 sprigs of Italian parsley

Heat the butter in a large pan and pan-fry the venison, turning it regularly for 5 minutes.

Mix in the flour and juniper berries. Add the garlic, bay leaves, thyme, and onions. Stir well, add the wine, mushrooms, carrots, and parsley root. Stir well again and let simmer for 20–25 minutes or until tender. The time it takes to get the meat just tender can vary a lot, so keep an eye on it, and take it off the heat when it is just right. Season to taste with salt and pepper.

Serve with the boiled potatoes, garnished with the parsley.

CELERIAC, a variety of celery grown specifically for its roots, makes a really good substitute for potatoes, but has fewer calories. It is very low in cholesterol, is a good source of fiber, vitamin B6, magnesium, potassium, and manganese, and is a very good source of vitamin C and phosphorus. Seeds are sown in February or March, planted out in May, and the root vegetable then comes straight from the fields from October to February.

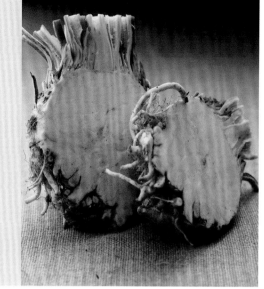

Mallard in apple cider with gingered red cabbage and celeriac mash

Mallard is a small duck with not a lot of meat on its carcass, but what meat there is can be very tasty and particularly nice with fall vegetables. SERVES 4

2 mallard ducks
generous 2 cups cider
2 bay leaves
1 tbsp whole peppercorns
salt

gingered red cabbage

½ red cabbage, shredded
3½ oz fresh ginger, minced
2 tbsp apple jelly (see page 126)
generous ¾ cup cider

celeriac mash

14 oz celeriac, peeled and
   cut into chunks
11 oz large potatoes, peeled and cut
   into chunks
2 tbsp extra virgin olive oil
salt and freshly ground pepper

Well ahead, cut each of the ducks in half lengthwise. Score some slashes in the skin through to the meat and put the duck halves in an ovenproof dish. Pour over the cider, add the bay leaves and peppercorns, and sprinkle with salt. Turn the birds so the meat is facing down and submerged in the cider. Cover with plastic wrap and let rest in the refrigerator until the next day or for at least 2 hours.

When ready to cook, preheat the oven to 350°F.

To make the gingered red cabbage: Place the cabbage in an ovenproof dish and mix in the ginger, apple jelly, and the cider. Place the ducks on top of the red cabbage, place in the preheated oven, and roast for 50 minutes. During that time, take it out of the oven twice and stir the red cabbage.

To make the celeriac mash: Cook the celeriac and potatoes in salted boiling water for 20 minutes or until tender, drain them, place them in a big bowl with the olive oil, and salt and pepper. Mash with a balloon whisk to a lumpy mash. Season again with salt and pepper to taste. Keep warm.

Carve the mallard meat and serve with the mash and red cabbage.

TIPS Instead of the mallard you can use duck breast or partridges.
Important: When you cook game, the cooking time can vary a lot according to the age of the animal/bird.

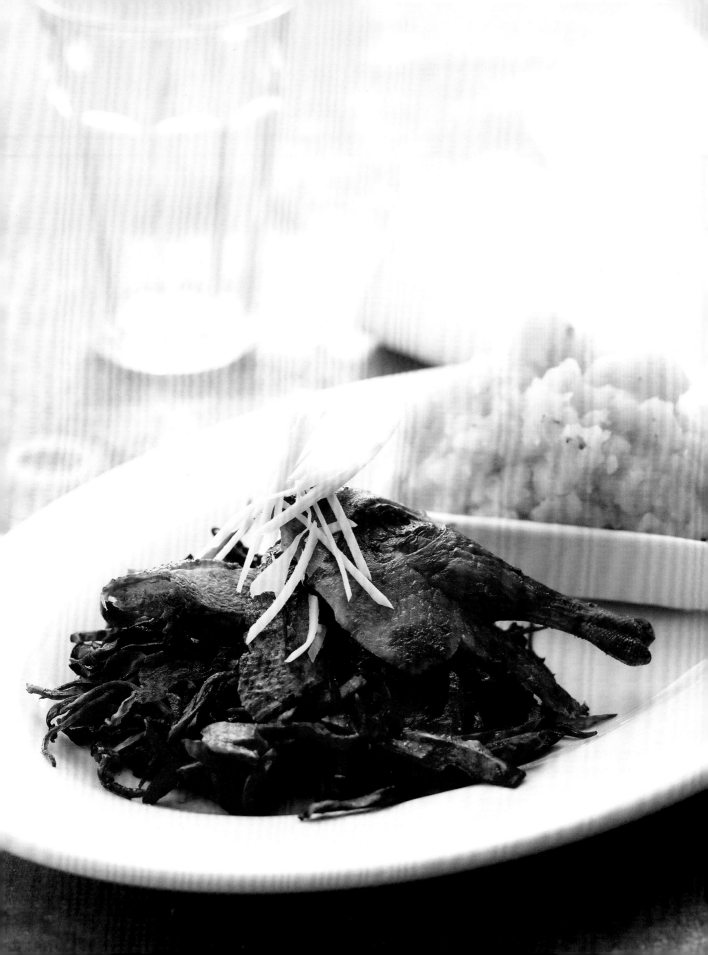

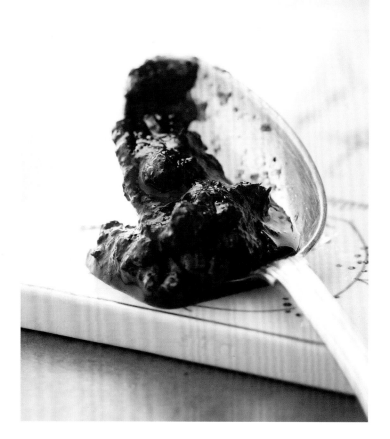

Leg of wild boar SERVES 10

1 leg of wild boar
6 garlic cloves, peeled
10 sprigs of rosemary
10 sprigs of thyme
2 tbsp salt
freshly ground pepper
generous 2 cups red wine

lingonberry compote

2¼ lbs fresh or frozen lingonberries
  (you can also use cranberries)
3 cups sugar

vegetables

1 lb 2 oz turnips
1 lb 2 oz Jerusalem artichokes
1 lb 2 oz carrots
2¼ lbs potatoes

To make the lingonberry compote, cook the berries in a generous ¾ cup boiling water for about 8 minutes. Add the sugar and let it boil for another 8 minutes, skimming the surface. Store in sterilized preserving jars.

Preheat the oven to 475°F. Start by preparing the boar leg: Cut off and discard a lot of the fat on the top. Then, with a small knife, cut slits deep into the meat and push the garlic down into them. Roughly chop both the rosemary and thyme sprigs, mix with the salt, and rub the leg with the herb mixture. Place in a big ovenproof dish and sprinkle with pepper.

Place in the preheated oven. After 10 minutes, turn the oven down to 325°F, add the wine, and 1¼ cups water, cover, and let braise for 2 hours. Should it dry up at any time, add a little more water.

Peel all the vegetables and cut them into chunks. Sprinkle with salt and pepper. After the boar has had an hour in the oven, take it out, place the vegetables under the boar, and put back in the oven for another hour.

After the 2 hours, check with a meat thermometer; if the meat is done, it should have an interior temperature of 176–185°F.

Serve the boar cut into thin slices, with the vegetables and lingonberry compote. And, if you like a salad, serve with the Kale salad on page 97.

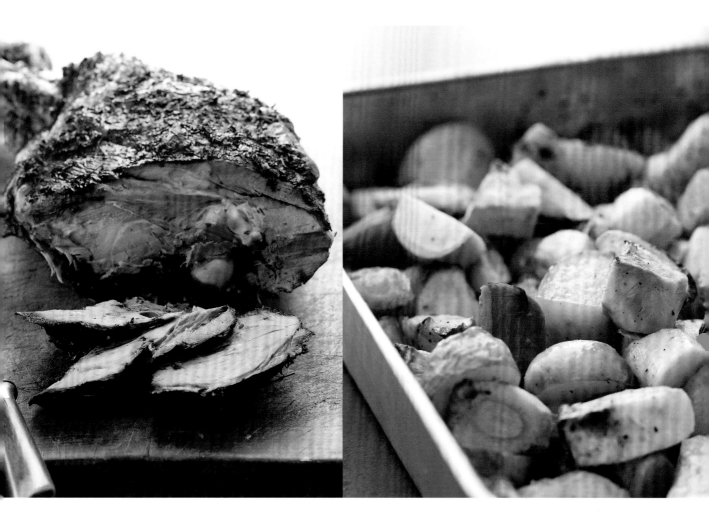

In Denmark, the hunting season for boar is all year round. You go into the woods around midnight and find a spot on a little hillock, then sit completely still, waiting for them. Sometimes they start coming in hordes and you need to sit completely still in order to assess the situation, finding out which is the perfect animal as, for example, you can't kill a mother or pregnant animal. Wild boar might not be low in calories, but there has to be room for feasts. It's all about striking a balance—intersperse days with few calories and days with a higher calorie intake. Don't count calories, or even think about them; think about the food and how good it tastes.

Desserts and Drinks

In our increasingly busy lives, there has to be a time and a place for sweet and comforting food. I believe that homemade cakes are the best because, again, you control what is in what you eat. A lot of the chocolate bars and cookies that we buy are full of additives and high in calories. If you buy chocolate, stick to good-quality dark chocolate as you can't eat too much of it. On the plus side, dark chocolate contains vitamin K, iron, magnesium, and antioxidants.

Cold yogurt mousse with red currants

Desserts do generally contain a lot of calories . . . that is just the way it is, so don't eat them regularly, and certainly not while trying to lose weight. However, these yogurt mousses are low in calories. Most desserts and cakes unfortunately don't lend themselves to the making of low-calorie versions without ruining the result, so eat fresh fruit instead. SERVES 4

3 gelatin leaves, immersed in cold
   water for about 5 minutes
1¾ cups Greek yogurt (10% fat)
generous ⅓ cup whipped cream
3 tbsp honey, plus extra to serve
generous ⅓ cup red currants

Mix the yogurt, cream, and honey well in a bowl.

Lift the gelatin out of the water and heat it gently in a small pan. Let it rest for 2 minutes, then slowly pour the gelatin into the yogurt mixture. Add half the red currants and mix them in.

Pour into 4 serving glasses and set aside until the yogurt starts to set, then put in the refrigerator for 4 hours before serving.

Serve cold with more honey and the remaining fruit on top.

TIP You can make these the day before; they make a very nice dessert to serve at brunch.

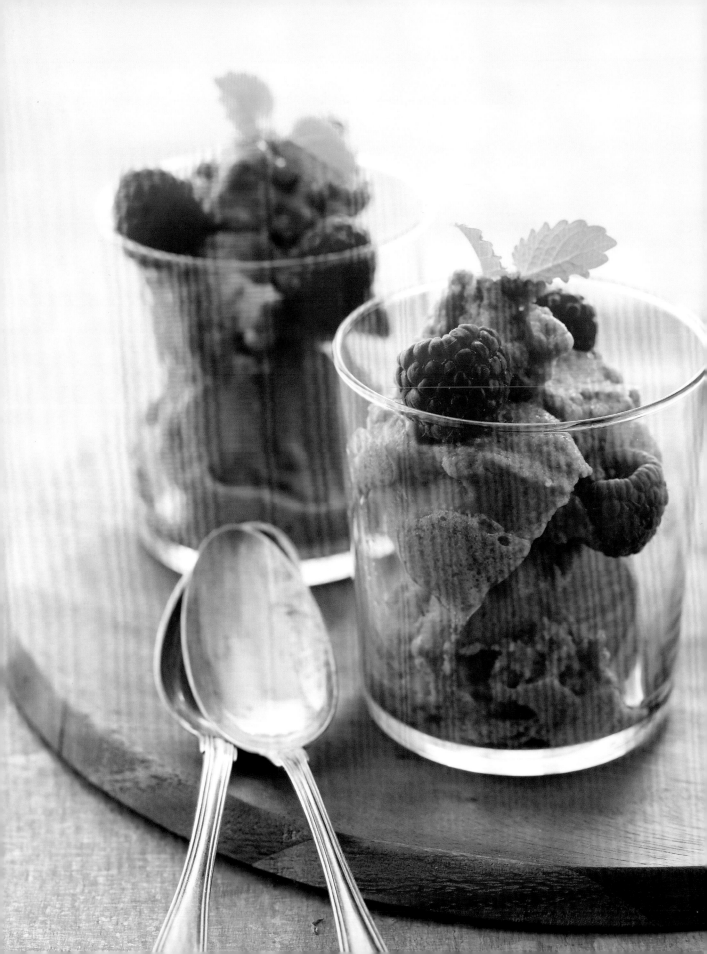

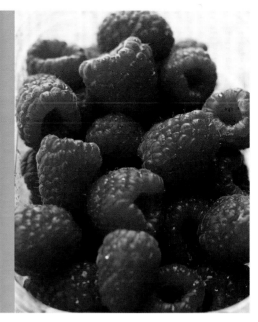

RASPBERRIES are members of the rose family and come in many colors apart from red: There are also black, purple, white, orange, and gold raspberries. They grow wild, and are cultivated, in the cooler parts of most of the northern hemisphere. Raspberries rank near the top of all fruits for antioxidant strength, particularly because of their dense content of ellagic acid, which is cancer-fighting. They are also very high in fiber and vitamin C, and a good source of magnesium, manganese, iron, and folate. In fact they are one of the richest sources in the human diet of manganese, a mineral which is necessary for correct bone growth and wound healing.

Raspberry lime sorbet

This sorbet is both palate cleansing and refreshing to eat—and also very easy to make. By making it yourself you can control the sugar content. Try experimenting to see how low you can go on the sugar and still love it! SERVES 4

1 cup sugar
3½ cups fresh or defrosted
  frozen raspberries, plus
  extra to serve
juice from 1 lime
mint leaves, to decorate

Mix generous 1 cup of water and the sugar in a pot, bring to a boil, lower the heat, and let it simmer for 3 minutes. Then chill this syrup.

Rinse the raspberries, dry them well, and then press them through a strainer so you have a raspberry puree without seeds.

Mix the raspberry puree with the syrup, a generous ¾ cup more water, and the lime juice. Taste to see if you need to add any more lime juice. Place in a plastic container and put in the freezer. Take it out 4 or 5 times every 15 minutes and stir thoroughly, then let it refreeze. Alternatively, use an ice-cream machine and, when finished, keep it in the freezer until you serve it, decorated with extra raspberries and mint leaves.

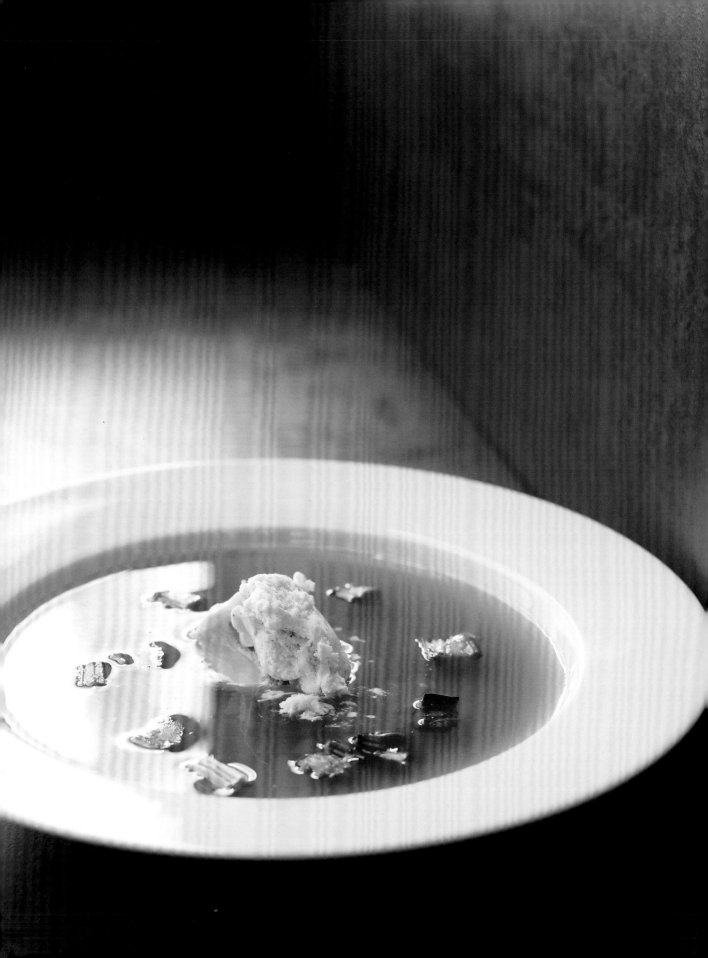

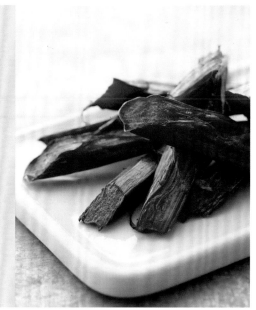

RHUBARB was cultivated in China for medical purposes more than 4,000 years ago. The stalks are rich in vitamin C, dietary fiber, potassium, and calcium, although the calcium is not easily absorbed by the body as it combines with the oxalic acid also in the plant. This problem can be minimized by cooking the rhubarb with angelica, which at the same time will reduce the amount of sugar needed. There are many varieties of rhubarb, some green, some red, some sour, and some sweet. Two good types are strawberry rhubarb and Victoria. The plant is perennial and very easy to grow, and its season is from March to May, although forced varieties can appear earlier.

Rhubarb soup with yogurt ice cream

This cold soup is perfect for a warm early summer day. Avoid bought vanilla sugar, which is usually just a chemical cocktail; instead, rinse a used vanilla bean and let it dry until stiff, then put it in a jar of sugar for a few days. SERVES 4

1½ lbs rhubarb
2 angelica stalks
1 vanilla bean
generous 1–1¼ cups sugar

baked rhubarb
2 rhubarb stalks, cut into
   ½-inch pieces
¼ cup sugar

yogurt ice cream
1¾ cups low-fat yogurt
¼ cup homemade vanilla sugar
generous ¾ cup whipping cream

At least 8 hours ahead, make the ice cream: Beat the yogurt and sugar together until the sugar is dissolved. Whip the cream until it forms soft peaks and fold it into the yogurt. Freeze in an ice-cream machine. If you don't have an ice-cream machine, pour it into a bowl and put it in the freezer for at least 6 hours, but stir it two or three times during that time.

Make the soup: Cut the rhubarb and the angelica into ¾-inch pieces and place in a pan. Add water to cover. Split the vanilla bean lengthwise and scrape out the seeds with a tip of a knife. Add these and the whole vanilla bean to the rhubarb. Bring to a boil, turn down the heat, and let simmer for 30 minutes. It is important that you do not stir it at all, otherwise the rhubarb will break up.

Line a strainer with cheesecloth and strain the cooked rhubarb through it. Return the strained liquid to a clean pan. Add the sugar and let it boil, stirring so that the sugar dissolves. Pour into a bowl and let it cool down.

When it has cooled, cover it and place it in the refrigerator until ice cold.

Make the baked rhubarb: Preheat the oven to 300°F. Place the rhubarb stalks in an ovenproof dish and sprinkle the sugar over it. Bake in the preheated oven for 30 minutes. Take out and let cool down.

Serve the cold soup with the rhubarb and the ice cream in the middle.

TIP If you don't have angelica you need to use about ½ cup more sugar.

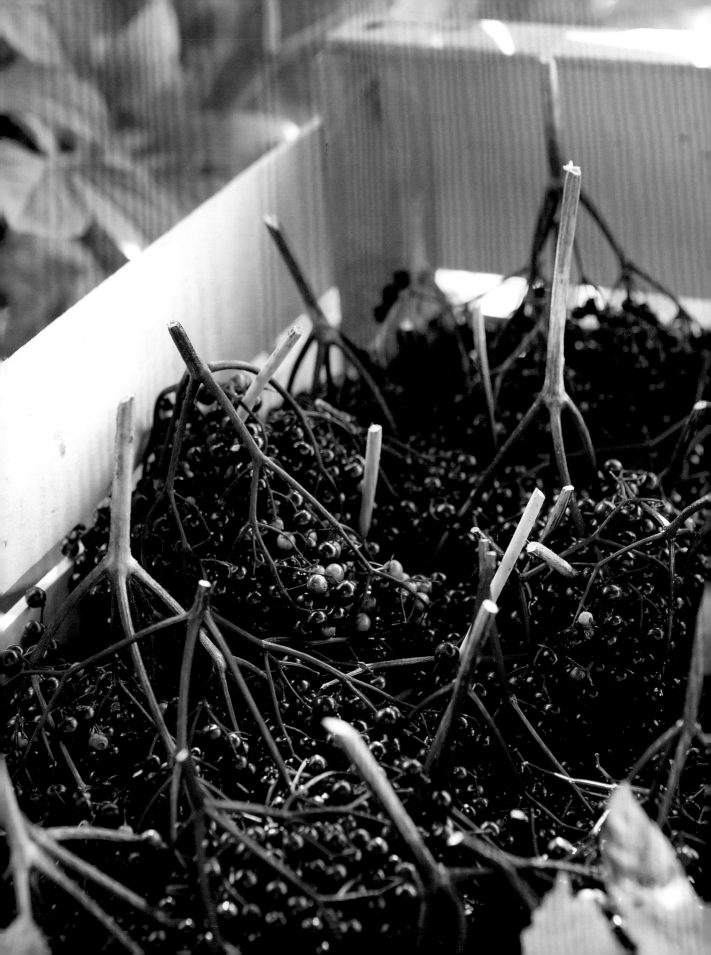

Elderberry soup with rye bread croutons

As a child I had this soup for dinner, but nowadays fruit soup is either served as a dessert or forgotten completely. It does, however, make a filling meal, and can be served as an afternoon snack or as a dessert. My mother would serve elderberry soup if we had a cold or a fever, and the grown-ups would drink hot elderflower punch with rum in it. SERVES 4

generous 2 cups elderberry cordial
  (see page 124)
1 tbsp cornstarch
1½ tbsp butter
3 slices of rye bread,
  cut into small cubes
2 apples, cut into slices

In a pan mix the cordial with a generous 2 cups water and bring to a boil.

Dissolve the cornstarch in a small amount of water, then stir it into the soup and slowly bring to a boil.

Melt the butter in a skillet and toss the rye bread cubes in it for 2–3 minutes. Let them rest on a plate.

Pour the soup into serving bowls and top with raw apple slices and rye bread croutons. Make sure the soup is served very warm.

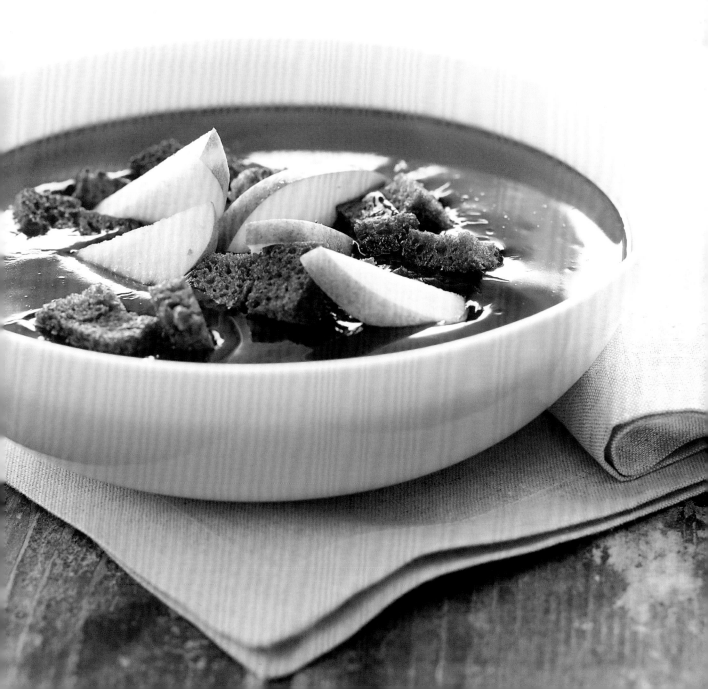

APPLES originate from central Asia, but are now grown worldwide. The fruits mature in fall. There are literally hundreds of varieties and their nutritional profile does vary wildly from one variety to another. They are high in antioxidant vitamin C and potassium, which is important in the metabolism of protein. They also contain the phytochemical quercetin which helps lower blood cholesterol levels. They have a low glycemic index so their use as a snack keeps hunger under control for longer than is the case with most other fruits.

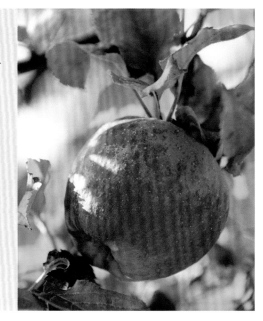

Apple and pear crumble with oats and cinnamon

In the fall I make this afternoon cake that is perfect with tea. I am sure that it is pretty healthy as there is very little sugar in it, and it contains both fiber and heaps of vitamins. When I serve it with yogurt instead of whipping cream, it is because I don't really care for whipping cream—I have always preferred yogurt or low-fat crème fraîche to cream. Try it, it is very refreshing! SERVES 8–10

3 pears (about 14 oz)
3 apples (about 1¾ lbs)
2¾ cups oats
½ cup raw organic sugar
⅔ cup almonds, coarsely
  chopped
2 tbsp ground cinnamon
4 tbsp butter, plus extra to grease
1¾ cups Greek yogurt, to serve

Preheat the oven to 400°F.

Cut the apples and pears in chunks, keeping the peel on but discarding the cores. Butter an ovenproof dish about 12 x 16 inches with straight sides. Place the fruit in the prepared dish.

In a mixing bowl, mix the oats, sugar, almonds, and cinnamon. Divide this mixture evenly over the fruit and then place small dots of butter all over the top. Bake for 30 minutes.

Serve warm with Greek yogurt.

TIP You can replace the apples and pears with plums or any fruit in season.

Oats, although having hardly any gluten, contain more antioxidants than wheat, as well as more soluble fiber than any other grain. Some of this fiber, known as beta-D-glucans, is believed to lower cholesterol in the human blood by up to 20 percent. Oats are also very high in protein (and the only cereal to have its protein in the same form as legumes), while they are low in saturated fat and very low in cholesterol and sodium. They are also a good source of thiamin, magnesium, and phosphorus, and a very good source of manganese. Grown in areas with cool, wet summers, such as northwest Europe, oats have a high natural oil content that gives them an extra lightness.

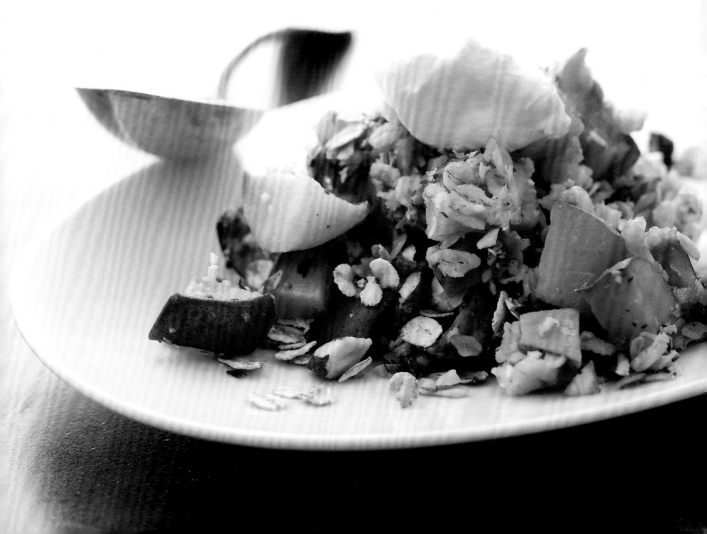

Strawberries contain large amounts of vitamin C (¾ cup has twice the daily recommended amount for adults) and the important vitamin K, which is needed for our blood to clot when we are wounded and for both bone and brain health. They also contain the phytochemical ellagic acid, which is known to fight the growth of cancer cells. Strawberries both grow wild and are widely cultivated throughout temperate parts of Europe and the United States. There are a huge number of varieties in various shapes and sizes; older ones, in particular, have a very intense taste, which to most northern Europeans instantly evokes that summer feeling.

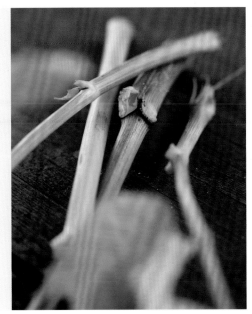

ANGELICA, a biennial Arctic plant, is very popular as a vegetable in Greenland. The Vikings found it on their expeditions there, noticing that people didn't suffer from scurvy although they were living in a harsh climate where very little can grow. They took the plant home, and angelica became the most important vegetable at that time in Denmark. In the Middle Ages, it was used as a medicinal herb and was one of the most important remedies against the plague. Use only stems from cultivated plants; don't pick them wild, as they are easily confused with very toxic giant hogweed. Angelica is very rich in vitamin C, and when cooked with vegetables containing oxalic acid it helps the body to absorb their calcium.

Rhubarb and strawberry tart

It is not always necessary to use a lot of sugar and fat to make a tasty dessert. Sometimes the natural flavors of the ingredients are sufficient. Skyr is an Icelandic cultured dairy product, somewhat like a soft cheese, that is high in protein and low in fat. It is suitable for breakfast, salad dressings, and desserts, or anywhere one would use yogurt. It is said to have been used by the Vikings, but is currently unique to Icelandic cuisine. SERVES 8–10

1 lb rhubarb, cut into ½-inch pieces
1 angelica stalk, cut into
½-inch pieces
1 vanilla bean
scant ¼ cup sugar
3½ cups strawberries, halved or
quartered
generous ¾ cup crème fraîche, to serve

pie dough
scant 1½ cups wheat flour
1 tbsp granulated sugar
scant ½ cup cold butter, cut into
small cubes
scant ½ cup quark or skyr

Make the pie dough: Sift the flour and sugar into a large bowl. Add the butter and rub in until the mixture resembles dry crumbs. Make a hollow in the middle and add the quark or skyr. Gather the dough with your hands to form a soft but not sticky ball. Wrap in plastic wrap and chill for 30 minutes.

Preheat the oven to 350°F and lightly butter an 11-inch round tart pan. Lightly flour the counter and roll the dough into a circle at least 14 inches in diameter. Use to line the tart pan and trim the edges by rolling the pin over the top of the pan, pressing down to cut off the excess dough.

Cover the dough with a circle of baking parchment and weigh it down with dried beans or rice. Bake blind for 15 minutes, then remove the paper. Bake for another 15–20 minutes until light brown and crisp. Cool on a wire rack.

Meanwhile, put the rhubarb and angelica in a pan. Split the vanilla bean lengthwise, scrape out the seeds, and mix with the rhubarb, then sprinkle with the sugar. Bring to a boil, cover, and simmer very gently for 20 minutes without stirring. Let cool. Spread the rhubarb in the tart case and cover with the strawberries. Serve with crème fraîche.

Cordial

I make cordial out of almost all types of berry. The uses for these cordials are innumerable: in salad dressings instead of honey; added to the cooking water when boiling root vegetables to give them extra sweetness; mixed with sparkling water to make sodas, which are much healthier than conventional ones as they contain less sugar and additives; poured over vanilla ice cream; diluted with water and frozen as popsicles; added to champagne for kir royale; topped off with boiling water for hot drinks in winter time. I also use cordials for hot punch with rum or cognac when I have a cold or a fever; this is way better than medicine.

Elderberry cordial
MAKES ABOUT 6⅓ CUPS

2¼ lbs elderberries
3 cooking apples, cut into quarters
2½ cups sugar

Rinse the berries, leave them on their stalks, but remove the coarse stalks. Place the berries and apples in a pot, add a generous 2 cups water, bring to a boil, and let simmer until the berries burst.

Line a strainer with cheesecloth and strain the cooked berries and apples through it. Put the resulting juice into a clean pot and bring to a boil. Add the sugar and let it boil for 2–3 minutes, skimming any scum from the surface. Pour the hot liquid into sterilized bottles. Store in your cupboard and, once opened, in your refrigerator.

Blueberry cordial
MAKES ABOUT 4 CUPS

2¼ lbs blueberries
1½ cups sugar

Rinse the berries, leave them on their stalks, but remove any coarse stalks. Put the berries in a pot, add a generous 2 cups water, bring to a boil, and let simmer until the berries burst.

Line a strainer with cheesecloth and strain the berries through it.

Put the resulting blueberry juice into a clean pan and bring to a boil. Add the sugar and let boil for 2–3 minutes, skimming any scum from the surface.

Pour the hot liquid into sterilized bottles. Store in your cupboard and, when opened, in your refrigerator.

Red currant cordial
MAKES ABOUT 4 CUPS

2¼ lbs red currants
1¾ cups sugar

Rinse the berries, leave them on their stalks, but remove the coarse stalks. Place the berries in a pot, add a generous ¾ cup water, bring to a boil, and let it simmer until the berries burst.

Line a strainer with cheesecloth and strain the berries through it.

Put the resulting red currant juice into a clean pan and bring to a boil. Add the sugar and boil for 2–3 minutes, skimming any scum from the surface.

Pour the hot liquid into sterilized bottles. Store in your cupboard and, when opened, in your refrigerator.

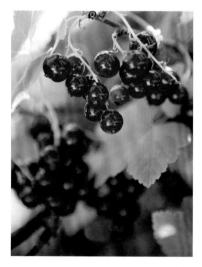

Shaken red currants

Serve this with chicken, fish, or any game during the summer. You can also serve it with your oatmeal in the morning or on yogurt.

2 cups red currants, stalks removed
1 cup sugar

Rinse the red currants in cold water, then drain them well.

Place them in a big tray and sprinkle with sugar. Shake the tray from time to time until the sugar has dissolved; it will take a couple of hours.

When the sugar has dissolved, pour the currants into a sterilized preserving jar and keep it in the refrigerator. They will keep for about 3 weeks.

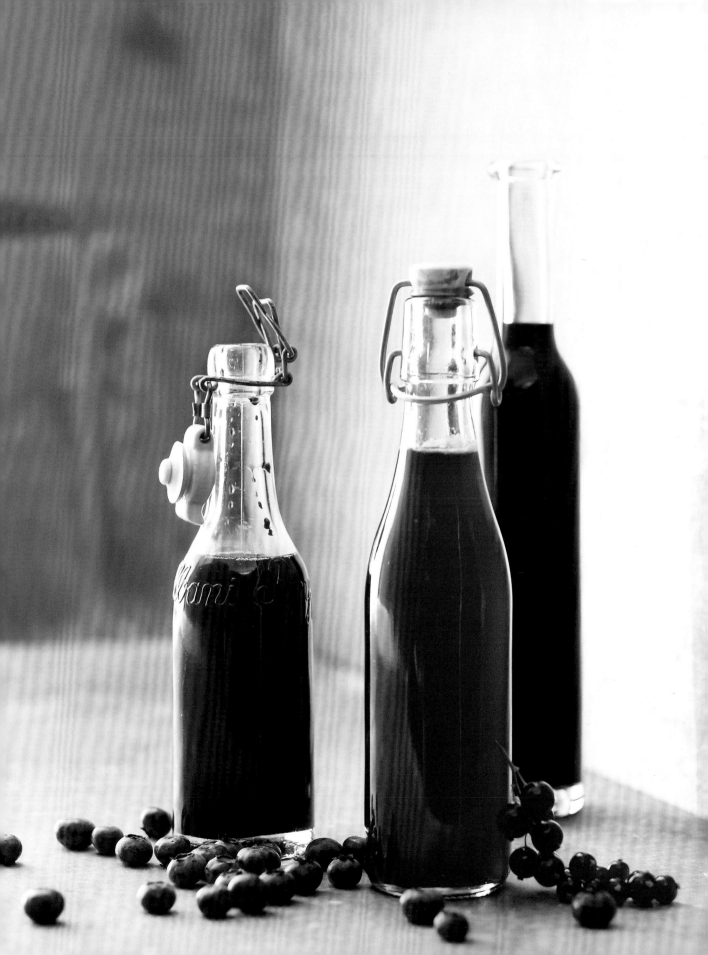

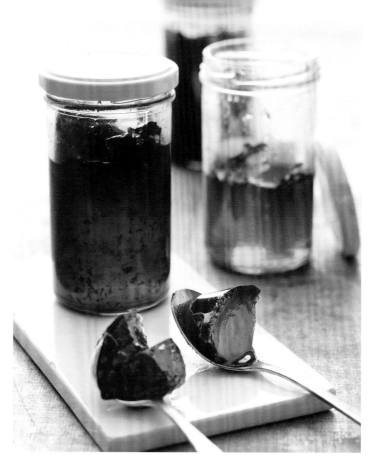

Apple jellies

Crab apple jelly
MAKES 5–6 ¾ CUP JARS

2¼ lbs crab apples
sugar (see below)

Cut the apples in half and put in a large pan. Add a generous 2 cups water and bring to a boil. Cover and simmer for half an hour. Strain the apples through a fine fabric and let drain until the next day.

Measure the juice and bring to a boil. Add 3¾ cups sugar per 4 cups of strained juice and simmer, uncovered, until some drops of the juice stick to the back of a spoon. Skim off any scum and pour the jelly into sterilized jars. Seal the next day.

Stored in a cold place, it will keep for months.

Mint apple jelly
MAKES 5–6 ¾ CUP JARS

2¼ lbs cooking apples
5 oz fresh mint leaves
sugar (see below)

Cut the apples into pieces, complete with peel and core. Put in a large pan. Add generous ¾–1¼ cups water, bring to a boil, cover, and simmer for 45 minutes. Don't stir at any time! Add the mint for the last 5 minutes.

Strain through a fine fabric and let drain until the next day. Measure the juice, bring to a boil, and add 4 cups sugar per 4 cups. Simmer, uncovered, until drops stick to the back of a spoon.

Skim off any scum and pour into sterilized jars. Seal the next day. Can be stored for months in a cold place.

Rowanberry and crab apple jelly
MAKES 5–6 ¾ CUP JARS

1 lb 2 oz rowanberries, destalked
1 lb 2 oz crab apples
sugar (see below)

Cut the apples into halves. Place in a pan, add 1¼ cups water, and bring to a boil. Reduce the heat, cover, and simmer for 30 minutes. Don't stir!

Strain the fruit through a fine fabric and let drain for 2–3 hours.

Measure the juice and add 2¼ lbs sugar per 4 cups of strained juice. Let it simmer, uncovered, until some drops stick to the back of a spoon.

Pour into sterilized jars and seal the jars the next day.

TIP If you prefer, use cooking apples.

ROSE HIPS, the fruit of wild and cultivated roses, contain large amounts of antioxidant vitamin C. They are also a good source of vitamins E and K, calcium, and magnesium, and a very good source of fiber, vitamin A, manganese, and omega-3 fatty acids. Pick them from late August to early September.

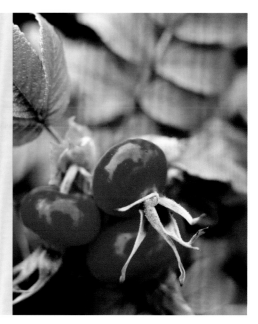

Rose hip syrup MAKES ABOUT 4 CUPS

1 lb 2 oz rose hips
generous ⅓ cup lemon juice
1¼ cups sugar

Cut the rose hips in half and remove the seeds with a teaspoon (use disposable gloves for this, as the seeds cause itching).

Place the rose hips, a generous 1 cup water, and the lemon juice in a pan, bring to a boil, and let it simmer, stirring occasionally, until very soft.

Pour into a jelly bag suspended over a bowl. Let drain overnight. Don´t press the bag or the juice will be cloudy.

Next day pour the juice into a pan, add the sugar, and bring to a boil. Let it boil until the juice has reduced by about half and is beginning to thicken. If necessary skim the syrup.

Pour the syrup into a sterilized bottles and seal.

Rose hip jam MAKES ABOUT 4 CUPS

2¼ lbs rose hips
2 small organic lemons
2 cups sugar

Cut the rose hips in half and remove the seeds (see left), then cut them into small pieces with a knife or in the food processor.

If you don´t have a zester tool, cut strips of the peel from the lemons with a vegetable peeler, leaving the bitter pith behind. Cut the strips into very thin julienne strips. Squeeze the juice from the lemons.

Combine the rose hips and a generous 1 cup water in a pan and bring to a boil. Cook for 15 minutes, then add lemon zest and juice, and the sugar. Stir to dissolve, then bring to a boil and maintain a full rolling boil for 10 minutes more, stirring frequently. Skim off any scum and let cool for 10 minutes.

Pour into sterilized jars and seal them. Store the jam in a cold place.

Breads

Homemade bread is one of the principal things that will help you when changing your diet. Factory-made bread is often full of calories, sugar, salt, and other additives. This is one of the reasons a lot of different diet movements have hit a chord by telling us that bread isn't healthy. Almost as important, though, is what industrial breads don't contain; only a small percentage use the whole grain, with all the fiber, nutrients, and slow-release energy that these impart. On the other hand, homemade bread, using different kinds of wholegrain flours and without a lot of added fat and sugar, is healthy and should be part of your daily diet. Not a whole loaf, mind you, but one or two slices a day. Baking your own bread gives you back control over what you eat, and it is not difficult at all if you build it into your routine.
I spend about 2 hours a week making bread dough and baking; the rest of the time it takes care of itself.

Rye syrup bread

This is a soft bread with a sweet taste. It is perfect with cheese and in the mornings, either freshly baked or toasted.
MAKES 2 LOAVES

2 oz yeast
generous 2 cups lukewarm water
¼ cup grapeseed oil
generous ⅓ cup light corn syrup
1 tsp salt
4 cups rye flour
scant 3 cups all-purpose flour

In a large mixing bowl, dissolve the yeast in the lukewarm water, then add the oil, syrup, salt, and flours. Stir together then knead; the dough should be firm but a bit wet. Leave under a dishtowel to rise for 45 minutes.

At the end of this time, divide the dough into 2 pieces and let rise again for 30 minutes, then place into the baking pans.

Preheat the oven to 350ºF and bake the loaves for 1 hour.

Let them cool on a wire rack.

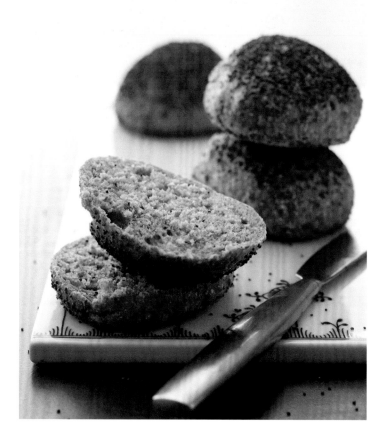

Rye buns

Buns can be served for breakfast, lunch, and as snacks, but this dough can also be made into a large loaf that is baked for 40 minutes. MAKES 20 BUNS

2 oz fresh yeast
1¾ cups yogurt
4 tbsp honey
¾ cup spelt flour
5 cups rye flour
scant 1½ cups all-purpose flour
1 tbsp salt
1 egg, beaten, to glaze
poppy seeds, to sprinkle

In a bowl, dissolve the yeast in 1¾ cups water and add the yogurt and honey. Mix the spelt flour, rye flour, all-purpose flour, and salt, and stir into the yeast mixture for about 5 minutes. On a floured counter, knead this dough well.

Place the dough back into the bowl, cover with a paper towel, and let rise at room temperature for about 1 hour.

Preheat the oven to 400ºF and line some cookie sheets with baking paper.

As the dough is a bit sticky, dust your hands with flour and form about 20 small buns from the dough with your hands. Place the buns on cookie sheets lined with baking paper. Glaze the buns with beaten egg and sprinkle with poppy seeds.

Bake the buns in the preheated oven for 30 minutes. When they are done, let them cool on a wire rack.

TIP Buns will last for 3–4 days, and are also very delicious when toasted. Remember never to store your bread in the refrigerator, as it will make the bread dry. Instead, store it in a dark, cool cupboard or breadbox.

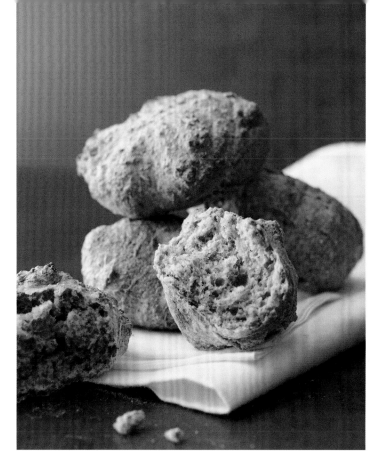

Shower buns

This recipe allows you to have homemade buns for breakfast during the week without any hassle! The biggest bonus is that you get healthy, tasty, homemade bread! It takes no time at all to place the buns on a cookie sheet and put them in the oven. They will be done when you come out of the shower. Not only do they taste wonderful, they will give your house that reassuring smell of home-baked bread in the morning. MAKES 14–16 BUNS

¼ oz (1 scant tbsp) yeast
1 tsp salt
1 tsp honey
generous 1¾ cups all-purpose flour
generous 2¾ cups spelt flour

The night before (or for at least 6 hours ahead): In a big bowl, mix the yeast into 2½ cups cold water, then add the salt and honey. Mix in the flours and give a good stir using a wooden spoon as it is a very soft dough. Cover the bowl with plastic wrap and place in the refrigerator overnight.

Next morning: Preheat the oven to 425°F. Cover a cookie sheet with baking paper and, using 2 spoons, mold the buns and place them on the cookie sheet. Bake in the oven for 20 minutes.

Take your shower after you have put the buns to cook; they will be ready for breakfast when you are! The buns should be golden and properly baked all the way through. A way to test this is to knock the base of a bun with the tip of your finger; the sound is hollow when the buns (or loaf) are done.

Let the buns rest on a wire rack for 5 minutes before serving for breakfast. Repeat every morning until there is no more dough.

Serve the buns with cheese, the strawberry jam on page 138, or a banana.

TIP Soft dough gives flat but moist buns. A firmer dough makes buns that rise higher but are less moist.

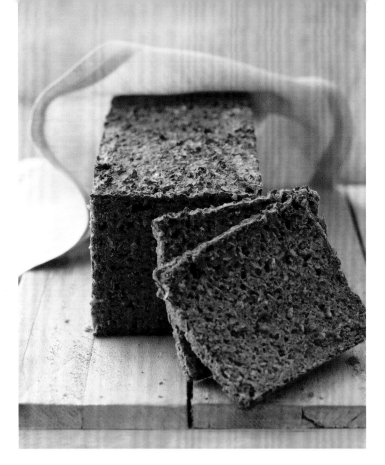

Rye bread

A friend of mine gave me a sourdough starter with this recipe more than twenty years ago, and the rye bread is still going strong. The sourdough has been through different crises over the years, where I have had to add a little salt, yeast, or buttermilk. It has traveled across the North Sea and the Atlantic Ocean when we lived in the UK and the United States. MAKES 1 LARGE LOAF

step 1: sourdough culture

scant 2¼ cups rye flour
1¼ cups buttermilk
1 tsp coarse sea salt

Mix the ingredients in a bowl. Cover with foil and leave for 2 days in a warm place (77–86°F). Then you have a sourdough culture! (If the temperature is too low, the sourdough will not develop but go bad.)

step 2: making the dough

3 cups lukewarm water
1 tbsp sea salt
3⅔ cups rye flour
2¾ cups wheat or fine spelt flour

In a large bowl, dissolve the culture from step 1 in the water. Then add the salt and the flours, and stir the dough with a wooden spoon. It should be a runny dough.

Cover the bowl with a towel and set aside for 12 hours at room temperature. I do it around dinnertime, then I can do step 3 the next morning.

step 3: making the bread

generous 1 cup lukewarm water
2 tsp salt
1 lb 2 oz cracked whole rye

Add the water, salt, and rye to the dough and stir again with a wooden spoon. Give it a good stir so all the rye grains are equally divided.

Remember every time you make the bread to take 3 tablespoons from the dough and mix it with 2 tablespoons coarse salt; save this in a container as your starter culture for the next time. Store it in the refrigerator and it will keep for up to 8 weeks.

Pour the dough into a 3¼-quart loaf pan. (If it is not a nonstick loaf pan you need to brush the inside with oil.) Cover the pan with a paper towel and let the dough rise for 3–6 hours, or until it has reached the top of the tin.

Preheat the oven to 350°F. Bake the loaf for 1 hour 45 minutes. When done, take it out of the pan immediately and let it cool on a wire rack.

Crispbread

Eat crispbread as part of a snack with smoked salmon, or for breakfast, or with a salad for lunch. MAKES 10

2 oz yeast
generous 2 cups lukewarm water
scant 3 cups all-purpose flour
scant 4 cups rye flour
1 tsp crushed caraway seeds
1 tsp salt
scant ½ cup butter

In a mixing bowl, dissolve the yeast in the lukewarm water.

Mix the flours with the caraway seeds and salt. Cut the butter into small cubes and add to the flour. With your hands, crumble the butter into the flour, then add the yeast mixture and knead well on a floured counter.

Put the dough in a bowl, cover with a dishtowel, and let rise for 1 hour at room temperature.

Preheat the oven to 475°F. Roll the dough out in a little rye flour to a very thin sheet. Cut out about 10 big round crispbreads and then cut out a small hole in the middle of each. Prick the crispbreads all over with a fork.

Place on cookie sheets and bake for 5–7 minutes, or until golden brown.

Let them cool on a wire rack. Store in an airtight container to keep them crisp.

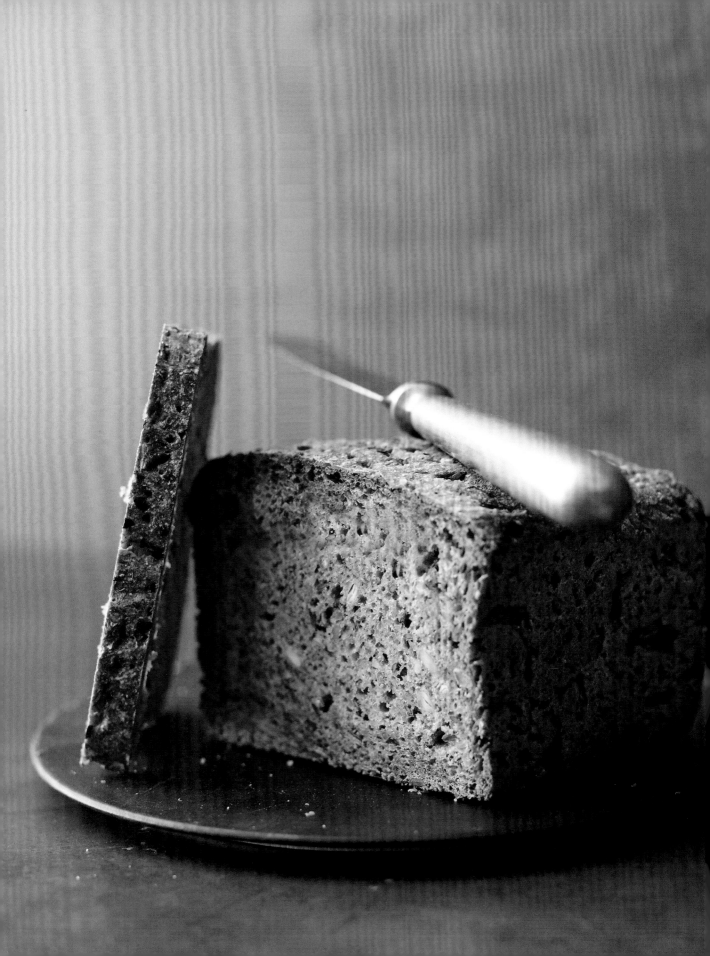

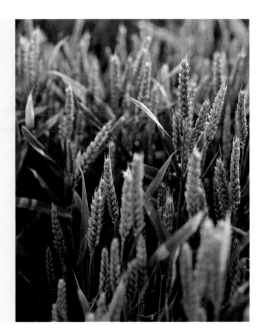

RYE contains more antioxidants and fiber than wheat, and less gluten. It is a good source of phosphorus and selenium, and a very good source of manganese. Rye also has a blood-cholesterol-lowering effect because it is rich in pentosans, a form of soluble fiber that helps inhibit the body's absorption of fat and cholesterol. Rye prospers in colder climates and poorer soils than wheat and is grown primarily in eastern, central, and northern Europe. When the water evaporates during the baking process, it risks making the rye bread very hard, and this is why rye flour is usually combined with sourdough and other types of flour in breadmaking.

Rye bread with flax seed and sunflower seeds

This rye bread has more seeds in it and therefore more calories, but it is extra healthy. MAKES 2 LOAVES

step 1: sourdough culture

⅓ oz yeast
generous ⅓ cup buttermilk
generous ⅓ cup (measure it by volume) wholewheat flour

Dissolve the yeast in the buttermilk. Mix the flour in well. Cover with foil and leave for 2–3 days at room temperature.

step 2: making the dough

3 cups lukewarm water
1 tbsp salt
11 oz cracked whole rye
¾ cup rye flour
generous ½ cup flax seeds
scant 2¾ cups wheat flour

Dissolve the culture in the lukewarm water. Add the salt, whole rye, rye flour, and flax seeds. Stir well, add the wheat flour, and stir again to a runny dough. Cover the bowl with a towel and set aside for 12–16 hours at room temperature.

step 3: making the bread

generous 1 cup lukewarm water
scant 4½ cups rye flour
scant ½ cup sunflower seeds

Add the lukewarm water and rye flour to the dough and stir well. Then take a generous ⅓ cup of the dough, put it in a glass container, sprinkle with coarse salt, cover with a lid, and store in the refrigerator. You now have a starter for the next time you make rye bread; it will keep for up to 8 weeks.

Add the sunflower seeds to the remaining dough and pour into 2 greased loaf pans (which together can contain 5½ lbs). Cover the pans with a dishtowel and let them rise at room temperature for 6 hours.

Preheat the oven to 350°F. Prick the dough with a knitting needle or fork and bake for 2 hours.

Let them cool on a wire rack.

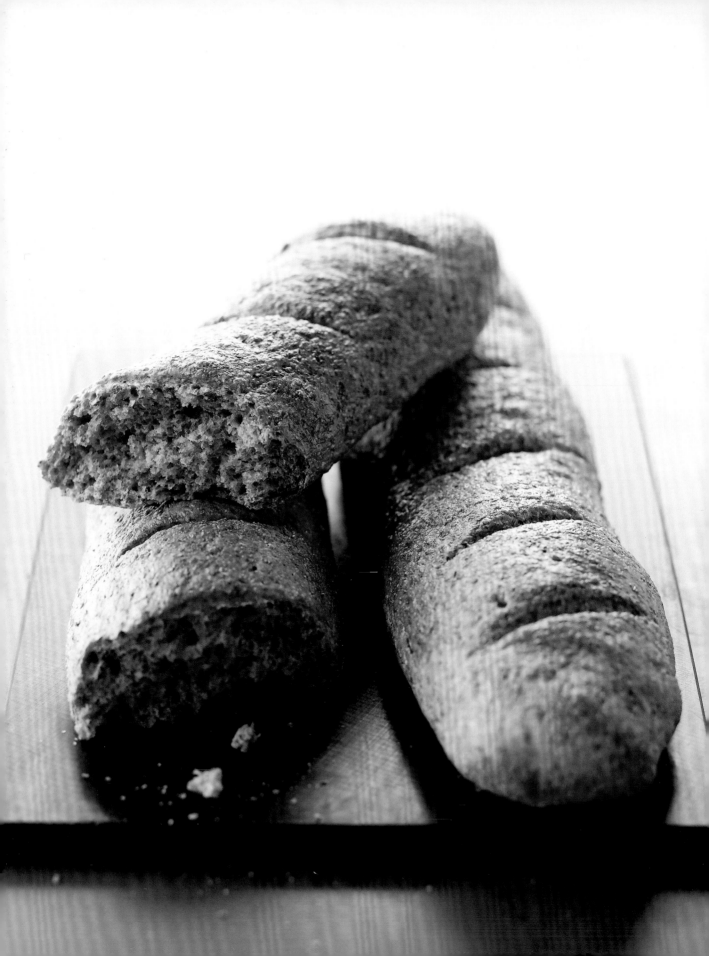

Spelt has more fiber and less gluten than ordinary wheat, but be sure to use coarse rather than fine spelt to get the full value of the fiber. The higher the fiber content, the better for digestion. Spelt is an ancient precursor of wheat and was a staple in medieval Europe before intensive plant breeding, but now has found a new market. It contains more nutrients than its commercial successors, and its natural yeasts and bacteria content also make it suitable for the production of a sourdough culture for breadmaking.

Spelt baguette

We all love baguettes and their associations with Paris. You can make your own, and you don't necessarily need to use only all-purpose flour. I make it with spelt as well. Instead of whole spelt flour, you can use wholewheat or rye flour.

MAKES 3 BAGUETTES

½ oz yeast
generous 2 cups lukewarm water
generous 1¾ cups all-purpose flour
3⅓ cups spelt flour
1 tbsp salt
1 beaten egg, for brushing

In a large mixing bowl, mix the yeast with 4 tablespoons of the lukewarm water. Add 2 tablespoons of the all-purpose flour and stir to a paste. Let rest under a dishtowel at room temperature for 20 minutes.

After the 20 minutes add the rest of the water and stir into the paste. Then add the remaining all-purpose flour and the spelt flour and the salt. Knead the dough well on a floured counter. Place in a big bowl and let rise under a dishtowel for 1 hour.

Divide the risen dough into 3 pieces and knead each lightly again. Form into 3 long baguettes, place on a greased cookie sheet, and let them rise again under a dishtowel for 20 minutes.

Preheat the oven to 425°F and place a little ovenproof bowl filled with water in the oven (this helps ensure a crunchy crust on the baguettes). Cut some small grooves on the surface of the dough, brush with egg, and bake in the preheated oven for 15 minutes. Lower the oven setting to 400°F and bake for 10 minutes more.

Take them from the oven and let them cool on a wire rack.

Serve the baguettes with soup, salad, lunch, or just as a snack with some cheese.

Spelt bread / Rhubarb and strawberry jam

If you bake your own bread, you control its contents completely, and then you know that it doesn't have a lot of sugar or additives, so why not do the same for your jam? Recipes for jam were more or less developed before the invention of the freezer and refrigerator, so all the berries had to be used when in season. To ensure that the jam lasted for the rest of the year, you had to conserve it with a lot of sugar, which you don't need to do when you can store the jam in a refrigerator. Jam can be fresher with little sugar; it then tends to have a wonderful, truer taste of the fruit. MAKES 1 LOAF

spelt bread

1 oz yeast

1 tbsp flaky sea salt

3 tbsp canola oil,
   plus extra to grease

1⅓ cups oats

3½ cups spelt flour

rhubarb and strawberry jam
(makes about 1¼ lbs)

1 whole vanilla bean

2 cups fresh or frozen organic
   strawberries

11 oz rhubarb, cut into small pieces

½ cup raw organic sugar

First make the jam: Split the vanilla bean lengthwise and place in a pan with the strawberries, rhubarb, and sugar. Bring to a boil and let boil for 15 minutes; if it dries out at any point, add a little water. Pour the hot jam into sterilized preserving jars and seal tightly. Store in the refrigerator.

Dissolve the yeast in a generous 2 cups cold water, then add the salt and oil. Mix again, then add the oats and flour and mix well for about 5 minutes.

Grease a 9½-inch diameter round baking pan or a 2-quart loaf pan with a little oil. Pour the dough into the baking pan and let rise in the pan for 4 hours and keep at room temperature.

Preheat the oven to 400°F and bake in the preheated oven for 1 hour. Let it cool on a wire rack.

Serve the bread with the jam (there's no need for butter as both bread and jam are so tasty).

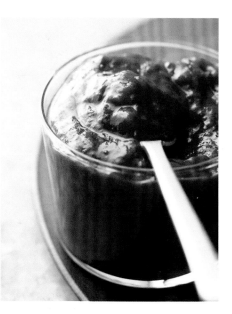

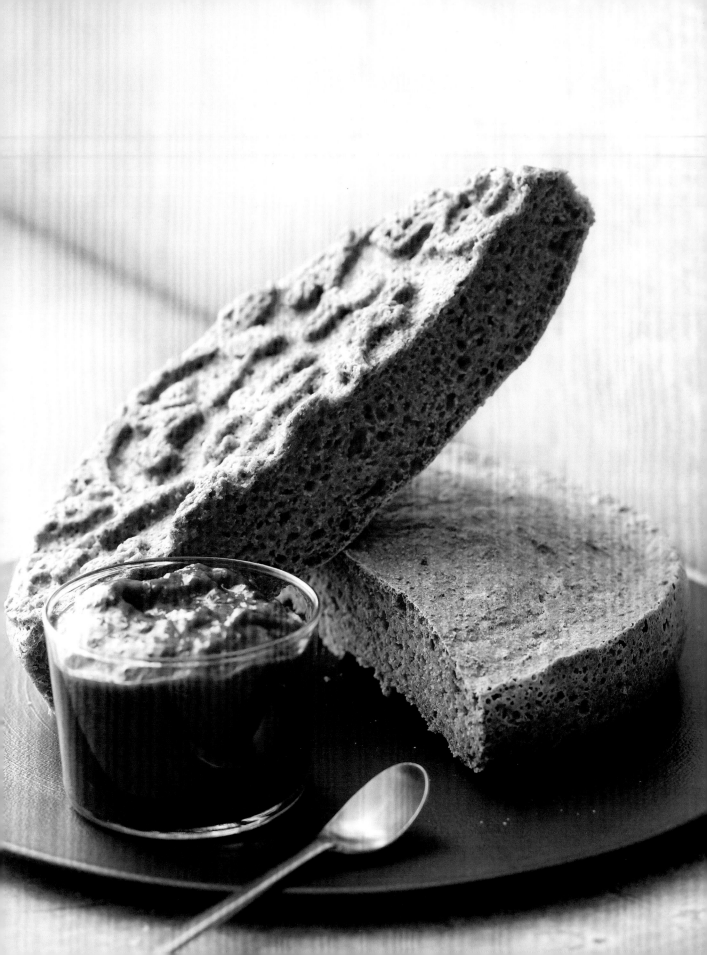

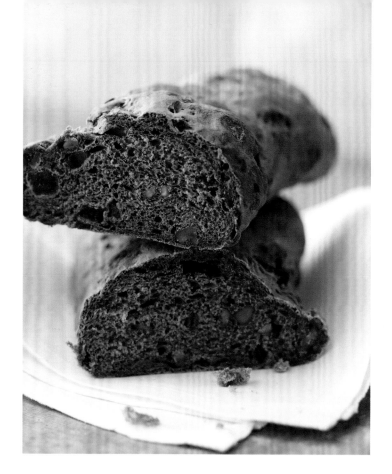

Malt bread with nuts and dried fruit

This is a lovely sweet and tasty bread speckled with nuts and dried fruit. It is very nutritious and very good with cheese. I have it with my afternoon tea. MAKES 2 LOAVES

2 oz yeast
2½ cups lukewarm water
generous ¾ cup low-fat yogurt
2 tbsp honey
2 tbsp malt flour
5¾ cups all-purpose flour
½ cup dried apricots, chopped
3½ oz dried dates, chopped
1 cup walnuts, chopped
2 tsp salt

In a large mixing bowl, dissolve the yeast in the lukewarm water, then add the yogurt and honey.

In a separate bowl, mix the flours, dried fruit, nuts, and salt. Stir this into the yeast mixture and mix well to an even and smooth dough.

Knead on a floured counter for 5 minutes. Place into a large bowl, cover with a dishtowel, and let rise for 1 hour.

Take the dough out of the bowl, form into 2 loaves, and place on a cookie sheet lined with baking paper. Cover with a dishtowel and let rise again for 30 minutes.

Preheat the oven to 400°F. After the 30 minutes' rising, bake the loaves in the oven for 40 minutes. Let them cool on a wire rack.

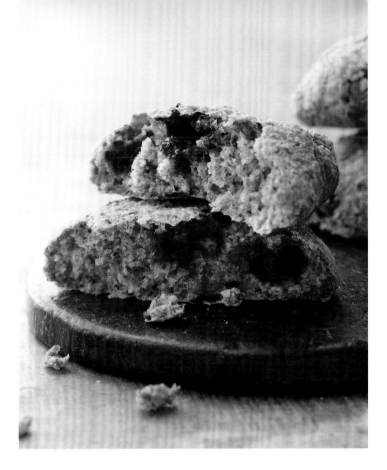

Blueberry buns

I use these sweet and nutty buns as "power snacks" to take with me when I go walking in the early morning on weekends.
MAKES ABOUT 20 BUNS

2 oz yeast
scant 3 cups lukewarm water
1 tsp salt
1 tbsp honey
1⅓ cups oats
3 cups wholewheat flour
scant 1½ cups all-purpose flour
scant ¾ cup blueberries
scant 1 cup coarsely chopped walnuts
scant 1 cup coarsely chopped hazelnuts

In a large mixing bowl, dissolve the yeast in the water, then add salt and honey together.

In another bowl, mix the oats and the flours, stir into the yeast mixture together with the blueberries, walnuts, and hazelnuts. Mix well with a wooden spoon. Knead the dough gently for a couple of minutes.

Cover with a dishtowel and let rise for 1 hour.

Form around 20 buns, place them on cookie sheets lined with baking paper, cover with towels, and let rise again for 30 minutes in a warm place.

Meanwhile, preheat the oven to 400°F. Glaze the loaves with water and bake in the preheated oven for 25–30 minutes. Let them cool on a wire rack.

Index

References

Maguelonne Toussaint-Samat, *A History of Food* (Blackwell, Oxford 1992)

Laura Stec with Eugene Cordero, *Cool Cuisine: Taking the Bite Out of Global Warming* (Gibbs Smith, Layton Utah 2008)

Judith Wills, *The Food Bible: The Ultimate Reference Book for Food and Your Health* (Quadrille, London 2007)

Paul Freedman (ed.), *Food: The History of Taste* (University of California Press, Berkeley 2007)

Ian Marber, *Supereating: A Revolutionary Way to Get More From the Foods You Eat* (Quadrille, London 2008)

Mark Bittman, *Food Matters: A Guide to Conscious Eating* (Simon and Schuster, New York 2009)

Judith Wills, *The Diet Bible* (Quadrille, London 2002)

Carolyn Steel, *Hungry City: How Food Shapes Our Lives* (Chatto & Windus, London 2008)

Acknowledgments

My thanks to my great team at Quadrille making this book, especially: Alison Cathie, Mark McGinlay, Claire Lattin, Anne Furniss, Helen Lewis, Nicola Davidson, and Lewis Esson—what an effort! Thanks to my agent Heather Holden Brown and Elly James for their encouragement and support. Also thank you to Lars Ranek for our fantastic collaboration—I really enjoy working with you.

Thanks to my fantastic kitchen team Lisa Høgh Nielsen, Anna Sofie Rørth, and Louise Lange for helping out in the kitchen, hours without end, inspiring me, and coming up with useful critical remarks. Thanks to my stepfather Henrik Rodam for foraging with me in the woods and teaching how to garden!

To my husband Niels Peter Hahnemann for all this support and long hours helping me writing the book. To my children Michala and Peter Emil for supporting me and eating recipes endlessly and coming up with critical responses.

10 9 8 7 6 5 4 3 2 1

Library of Congress Cataloging-in-Publication Data

Hahnemann, Trina.
  The Nordic diet : using local and organic food to promote a healthy lifestyle / Trina Hahnemann ; photography by Lars Ranek.
      p. cm.
  Includes bibliographical references and index.
  ISBN 978-1-61608-189-8 (pbk. : alk. paper)
  1. Reducing diets. 2. Reducing diets--Recipes. I. Title.
  RM222.2.H219 2011
  613.2'5--dc22
                                    2010031948

Printed in China